YOUR TYPE 2 DIABETES ACTION PLAN

Tips, Techniques, and Practical Advice for Living Well with Diabetes

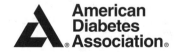

American Diabetes Association

Director, Book Publishing, Abe Ogden; *Managing Editor,* Greg Guthrie; *Acquisitions Editor and Editor,* Rebekah Renshaw; *Production Manager and Composition,* Melissa Sprott; *Cover Design,* Sport Creative; *Printer*, Data Reproductions.

Printed in the United States of America
1 3 5 7 9 10 8 6 4 2

The suggestions and information contained in this publication are generally consistent with the *Standard of Medical Care in Diabetes* and other policies of the American Diabetes Association, but they do not represent the policy or position of the Association or any of its boards or committees. Reasonable steps have been taken to ensure the accuracy of the information presented. However, the American Diabetes Association cannot ensure the safety or efficacy of any product or service described in this publication. Individuals are advised to consult a physician or other appropriate health care professional before undertaking any diet or exercise program or taking any medication referred to in this publication. Professionals must use and apply their own professional judgment, experience, and training and should not rely solely on the information contained in this publication before prescribing any diet, exercise, or medication. The American Diabetes Association—its officers, directors, employees, volunteers, and members—assumes no responsibility or liability for personal or other injury, loss, or damage that may result from the suggestions or information in this publication.

Jane Chiang, MD, conducted the internal review of this book to ensure that it meets American Diabetes Association guidelines.

∞ The paper in this publication meets the requirements of the ANSI Standard Z39.48-1992 (permanence of paper).

ADA titles may be purchased for business or promotional use or for special sales. To purchase more than 50 copies of this book at a discount, or for custom editions of this book with your logo, contact the American Diabetes Association at the address below or at booksales@diabetes.org.

American Diabetes Association
1701 North Beauregard Street
Alexandria, Virginia 22311

DOI: 10.2337/9781580405645

Library of Congress Cataloging-in-Publication Data
Your type 2 diabetes action plan : tips, techniques, and practical advice for living well with diabetes / American Diabetes Association ADA.
        pages cm
 Summary: "This book will help the reader discover how a diabetes care plan can help them take charge of diabetes"-- Provided by publisher.
 Includes bibliographical references and index.
 ISBN 978-1-58040-564-5 (paperback)
 1. Non-insulin-dependent diabetes. 2. Self-care, Health. I. American Diabetes Association.
 RC662.18.Y68 2015
 616.4'624--dc23
                        2015014065

Contents

Chapter 1

About Diabetes

Here, we'll dig into the basics of diabetes, including the roles of insulin and glucose. You'll find out about different types of diabetes and different people who have diabetes. In this chapter, you'll also learn about diagnostic tests and risk factors for you and your family. Most importantly, discover how a diabetes care plan can help you take charge of your diabetes.

WHAT'S INSIDE:

- What Is Diabetes?
- What Is Insulin?
- Insulin and Glucose
- Types of Diabetes
- Prevalence of Diabetes
- Diagnosing Diabetes
- Risk Factors for Type 2 Diabetes
- Diabetes Care Plan

WHAT IS DIABETES?

You've heard the word diabetes. Probably you or someone in your family or a friend has diabetes. But what does it really mean?

There are different types of diabetes, with type 1 and type 2 diabetes being the most common forms. Diabetes shares a common thread: the body's inability to make insulin or use insulin properly or a combination of both. OK, so insulin is a key player in diabetes, but what exactly *is* insulin?

WHAT IS INSULIN?

Insulin is a hormone that our body produces in the pancreas. We use insulin to do lots of amazing things in our bodies, but one of its main jobs is to help us convert the food that we eat into forms of energy that are "stored." Our body can use this stored energy later, when we might need it.

INSULIN AND GLUCOSE

Insulin does not work alone. In fact, insulin works closely with a sugar called glucose to make our bodies run smoothly. After we eat, our body turns that cinnamon raisin bagel or fish taco into smaller building blocks of nutrients. One of those building blocks is called glucose.

Glucose travels into our bloodstream to different cells. Here's the catch: our body needs insulin to help glucose get into some of the necessary cells. Without insulin, glucose can't do its job of saving energy for our bodies. Insulin and glucose work together to create stored energy, which is so essential for our bodies.

In diabetes, our body can't make or use insulin properly and things go awry. Stored energy may be broken down into *too much* fuel at a time when we don't need it.

TYPES OF DIABETES

There are several different types of diabetes, but the two most common types of diabetes are type 1 and type 2. Scientists distinguish the different types of diabetes by what tends to happen inside our bodies in terms of insulin and glucose.

In type 1 diabetes, your body destroys the cells in your pancreas (beta cells) that make insulin. Sometimes this destruction can happen quite quickly. This is why you may have heard about a child or adult rushed to the hospital and diagnosed with type 1 diabetes. Other times, the destruction occurs more slowly, such as in adults with latent autoimmune diabetes, called LADA. In general, people with type 1 diabetes cannot make enough insulin.

DIABETES WORLDWIDE

- Around the world, 382 million people had diabetes in 2013.
- Type 2 diabetes appears to be increasing in every country.

Source: International Diabetes Federation

In type 2 diabetes, your body may have problems with the beta cells that make insulin or problems with the cells that receive insulin to do their jobs—or both. In other words, your body doesn't make enough insulin and your body isn't as sensitive to insulin, or a combination. The good news is that many people with type 2 diabetes are able to boost their production or sensitivity to insulin by making healthy lifestyle changes or taking medications. Therefore, you can do something about your diabetes!

Some women get diabetes when they become pregnant, which is called gestational diabetes. It usually goes away after pregnancy, but you are more likely to have it with future pregnancies. Also, women with gestational diabetes are more likely to develop type 2 diabetes later. If you have gestational diabetes, you'll work with your health care provider to manage your diabetes during your pregnancy to keep you and your baby healthy.

Prediabetes

Some people have higher than normal blood glucose that is not high enough to be considered diabetes. It is called *prediabetes*. Half of Americans 65 and older have prediabetes, according to the Centers for Disease Control and Prevention (CDC). People with prediabetes may not have any symptoms. Yet, it's important to diagnose people with prediabetes because these people are at high risk for someday developing diabetes. And studies show that making changes to diet and exercise and even taking medication can delay diabetes in these patients.

PREVALENCE OF DIABETES

The vast majority of people with diabetes have type 2 diabetes. About 90 to 95 percent of people with diabetes have type 2, while 5 to 10 percent of people with diabetes have type 1.

You are not alone with your diabetes. In fact, over 9.3 percent of Americans have diabetes. That means 29.1 million people have diabetes in the United States, according to CDC estimates from 2014. These numbers are just estimates. We don't really know. In fact, many people *have* diabetes, but don't know it. Roughly 8.1 million or 27.8% of the 29.1 million people with diabetes in the U.S. are undiagnosed. Probably, if you're reading this book you have diabetes or know someone who has diabetes—and you want to do something about it.

Who Should Be Tested for Diabetes?

- Adults who are overweight with a body mass index (BMI) equal to or greater than 25 kg/m^2 or 23 kg/m^2 in Asian Americans and additional risk factors such as a family history of diabetes, not being active, high blood pressure, or a history of cardiovascular disease
- Anyone 45 years of age or older
- If negative, test should be repeated at least every 3 years

DIAGNOSING DIABETES

You may have heard the term blood glucose when you were first diagnosed. Your health care provider may have taken a blood sample and run a test on your blood that indicated that you have diabetes. There are several tests that providers use: A1C, fasting plasma glucose, two-hour plasma glucose, or random plasma glucose. Now, those are a mouthful. The important thing to remember is that all these tests give a measurement of the glucose in your blood. A higher amount of blood glucose indicates that you may have diabetes.

Tests for Diagnosing Diabetes

- A1C greater than or equal to 6.5
- Fasting plasma glucose greater than or equal to 126 mg/dL
- Two-hour plasma glucose greater than or equal to 200 mg/dL

- Random plasma glucose greater than or equal to 200 mg/dL in patients with symptoms of high blood glucose

Tests for Prediabetes

- Fasting plasma glucose 100–125 mg/dL
- Impaired glucose tolerance (2-hour plasma glucose after a 75-g oral glucose tolerance test of 140–199 mg/dL)
- A1C of 5.7–6.4

RISK FACTORS FOR TYPE 2 DIABETES

A1C

Short for Hemoglobin A1c. Hemoglobin is the part of our red blood cell that carries oxygen. When it attaches to glucose, it becomes "glycosylated." Scientists measure the amount of glycosylated hemoglobin to then give a picture of your average blood glucose over two to three months.

No one knows for sure what causes type 2 diabetes. Yet, we know that certain things put people at higher risk for diabetes: age, a family history of diabetes, being overweight, race and ethnicity, prediabetes, and having diabetes during pregnancy.

Age. Your risk of developing diabetes increases with age. Therefore, everyone 45 or older should be regularly tested for diabetes (every three years).

Family History. A family history of diabetes is a risk factor because people who have parents or siblings with diabetes are more likely to have diabetes themselves. Your father or mother or grandmother or grandfather may have passed on genes that put you at higher risk for diabetes. No one has found a "diabetes gene," and in fact, scientists imagine that a complex set of genes and interactions are at work.

Weight. Being overweight is also a risk factor for diabetes. People who are overweight cannot use insulin as effectively, which is called insulin resistance. The body tries to make up for this resistance by making more and more insulin to try to move glucose out of the blood and into cells. Over time, the pancreas sometimes cannot keep up and glucose in the blood rises. The shape of your body or where you carry extra weight can also be a risk factor for diabetes. For example, people with an "apple" body shape, in which you carry weight above your belt, are at higher risk for diabetes.

Race/Ethnicity. Your race and ethnicity also play a role in diabetes. African Americans, Latinos, Native Americans, and Asians are more likely to develop diabetes than non-Hispanic whites.

Prediabetes. Remember prediabetes from before? People with prediabetes are more likely to develop type 2 diabetes than people without prediabetes.

Gestational Diabetes. Women who had diabetes during pregnancy are seven times more likely to develop type 2 diabetes than women who did not have diabetes during pregnancy. Their babies may also have a higher risk for being overweight and developing type 2 diabetes when they grow up.

Blood Pressure. People with high blood pressure are more likely to have type 2 diabetes, so this is a risk factor as well.

Some risk factors are unchangeable: your family history, your race and ethnicity, your age. They're part of what makes you unique. Other risk factors are more changeable: your weight and blood pressure. Making changes in your lifestyle and health can reduce your risk for developing diabetes or help you live better with your diabetes for years to come.

DIABETES CARE PLAN

One of the keys is to come up with a plan for managing your diabetes. Together with your health care provider, you'll formulate a plan for taking care of you and your diabetes. This is called a diabetes care plan.

Your plan may include: checking your blood glucose, eating well, exercising, taking medications, and monitoring complications. It is unique and needs to fit you and your lifestyle: your age, your family life, your work, your current health, and your priorities.

You, the patient, are at the center of your diabetes care plan.

You may work with your primary care physician or a number of different health care providers to come up with your plan. They could include a physician, nurse practitioner, physician assistant, pharmacist, diabetes educator, or dietitian. The most important person in your plan is *you*. You'll need to take an active role to make sure you come up with the best plan that works for both your diabetes and your life.

NEXT UP

The following chapters outline important aspects of a diabetes care plan, including checking and managing blood glucose, lowering your blood pressure and cholesterol, food, exercise, medications, and complications. Next up: checking and managing blood glucose.

Chapter 2

Check and Manage Blood Glucose

In this chapter, find out about one aspect of your diabetes care plan: checking and managing your blood glucose. Why is this important? Keeping your blood glucose on target will minimize your risk for complications such as eye, kidney, and nerve disease. It may also help your mind and body feel better on a day-to-day basis—and everyone could use a little more of that.

WHAT'S INSIDE:

- Checking Blood Glucose
- A1C
- Blood Glucose Meters
- Continuous Glucose Monitors
- Basics of Self-Monitoring
- Hypoglycemia
- Hyperglycemia
- Sick Days
- Pregnancy

CHECKING BLOOD GLUCOSE

Checking your blood glucose is one of the best ways to keep track of your diabetes care plan. You can use the readings on your own and with your health care provider to monitor how different activities and situations affect your body. For example, exercise, food, medications, stress, and sickness can all affect your blood glucose. Monitoring is the only way to measure how these specific things impact you.

The two most common ways people check their blood glucose are: an A1C test and a handheld meter.

A1C

As mentioned in the last chapter, an A1C test is done in your health care provider's office or a laboratory using a sample of blood from your finger or vein. The A1C can be used to diagnose diabetes and it can also be used to manage your existing diabetes.

The test gives an average of your blood glucose over the past two to three months. It is a broad picture of how your diabetes care plan is working, and it can be an extremely useful tool for you and your health care provider.

In general, many people with type 2 diabetes will aim for an A1C below 7, which has been shown to reduce the risk of eye, kidney, and nerve damage, and heart disease. Some people may aim for a lower or higher A1C based on their age, how long they've had diabetes, and their general health.

HOW OFTEN TO TEST A1C

- At least two times a year for people meeting goals and keeping blood glucose on target
- Four times a year for people making changes to their plan or not meeting goals

BLOOD GLUCOSE METERS

A blood glucose meter allows you to check your blood glucose by yourself any time of the day. A meter displays your plasma glucose level, or the amount of glucose in your plasma as milligrams per deciliter (mg/dL).

Unlike the broad picture of an A1C, a reading from your meter gives you a specific snapshot of your blood glucose in that moment.

Meters come in many sizes and styles, with cool features. In general, you'll use a lancet to prick your fingertip and draw a small amount of blood. Next, you'll put the blood sample onto a test strip and insert it into the meter. The meter then displays your blood glucose reading. Your readings (usually 100 or more) are stored in the meter until you download them to your computer or write them down in a logbook.

Helpful Meter Features

- Size: Large displays may help people with poor eyesight, while small devices slip into a purse or pocket more easily.
- Strip Type: A pre-loaded drum of test strips may be easier to handle than individual strips.
- Bright Lights: For nighttime or dim light.
- Audio: Spoken readings and prompts ideal for those with vision problems.
- Size of Blood Drop: Smaller sizes are usually easier.
- Wireless Bluetooth Capacity: Deliver results wirelessly to phone or computer.
- Memory: Some can store thousands of readings.

PLASMA VS. WHOLE BLOOD GLUCOSE

Today, most meters measure plasma blood glucose. Years ago, meters used to display whole blood glucose. Plasma has more liquid and therefore more glucose, giving a higher percentage reading of glucose than whole blood. "Whole blood" is the liquid and the "cells" in the liquid. That's why today's blood glucose targets may appear higher than in previous decades.

Meters and Test Strips

Each meter comes with its own set of instructions and guidelines for maintenance. Read these carefully and call the toll-free number or talk to your health care provider if you have questions.

The chemical make-up of test strips varies slightly from batch to batch, so meters need to be calibrated to take these variations into account. Most meters calibrate themselves, which means that they reset themselves to ensure the most accurate reading. However, some meters may require that you calibrate for each new batch of test strips.

Control solution helps ensure that you're getting the most accurate readings. The solution contains a known amount of glucose so that you can run a test to make sure your meter and strips are working properly. Your meter should come with control solution or ask your pharmacist.

Test again if a reading is unexpectedly high or low—near the same site and making sure to get enough blood on the test strip.

Make sure that you use the recommended test strips for your meter. Using the wrong test strips could give you an incorrect reading. Test strips are vulnerable to temperature, moisture, and sunlight, so try to take care of your supplies (after all, they're not cheap). Close up the package after it's opened and keep it out of extreme temperatures like a backpack left in the sun or the glove compartment of your car on a freezing cold night. Note the expiration date on the package and be sure to throw away expired strips.

METER TIP

Wash hands with soap and water, and dry completely. Keep in mind, alcohol wipes and hand sanitizers can affect readings.

If you're having problems or trying a new meter, bring it to your next health care appointment to make sure you're using it correctly.

FDA Regulation of Meters

The U.S. Food and Drug Administration regulates blood glucose meters as medical devices. The FDA reviews the accuracy and consistency of meters before they can be marketed to consumers. The agency also relies on reports of problems from patients and health care providers to monitor the ongoing efficacy of devices once they're on shelves. If you suspect a problem with your meter or test strips, you can report it to FDA's Medwatch online or by calling 1-800-INFO-FDA.

WHAT IS EAG?

eAG is your estimated average glucose and is given in mg/dL—just like your meter. Your health care provider may test your eAG to help evaluate how your diabetes care plan is working.

CONTINUOUS GLUCOSE MONITORS

A continuous glucose monitor is a device that you attach to your body to take blood glucose readings throughout the day and night. It consists of three parts: a sensor with a needle that you insert under your skin, a transmitter, and a receiver to display and store readings. Continuous glucose monitors (CGMs) help you visualize how your blood glucose is trending—up or down—rather than just a moment in time like a finger prick with a meter. CGMs also have programmable alerts that beep when your blood glucose gets dangerously low or high. Most people who use CGMs have type 1 diabetes. Some people with type 2 diabetes may find them helpful, too.

BASICS OF SELF-MONITORING

Monitoring your blood glucose is all about gathering information—information that will help you take care of yourself. Your results may prompt you to eat a snack, exercise more or less, or discuss changes in your care with your provider. Monitoring may alert you to treat high or low blood glucose. And recording your results can help you and your health care team evaluate how different foods, exercise, and medications affect your blood glucose.

Blood Glucose Goals

Blood glucose goals are the foundation of your diabetes care plan. Your goals are the target ranges that you'll want to keep your blood glucose on a daily or longer-term basis. Blood glucose goals can vary tremendously from person to person. Someone who is first diagnosed with type 2 diabetes may aim for a broad target over three months while someone who has had type 2 diabetes for years may check their blood glucose five times a day.

Keeping Records

How you decide to record your blood glucose readings is up to you—and your health care provider. You may find it helpful to write down each reading in a notebook or chart. Or you may find it easier to export readings from your meter to a computer program like Excel or a website. You may do

ADA RECOMMENDATIONS FOR BLOOD GLUCOSE LEVELS

- A1C <7
- Before Meal: 80–130 mg/dL
- Post Meal (1–2 hours after beginning a meal) <180 mg/dL

Some patients may have different goals based on their age, how long they've had diabetes, other health conditions, or personal considerations.

NEW SOFTWARE AND APPS

New blood glucose apps, software, and websites are constantly being developed. Check out *Diabetes Forecast* magazine's annual consumer guide (January issue) for the latest technology or search iTunes for "diabetes."

it every day or once a week. You might be taking two or three readings a day or many more. Record keeping is individual, but it is also essential for most people with diabetes.

Visualizing how different activities and situations affect your blood glucose is the most import aspect of keeping records. Without records, you don't have solid data—just guesses. There are not "good readings" or "bad readings." It is simply a way to measure what may or may not be working best for you as part of your diabetes care plan.

Times to Check

Talk to your health care provider about the times to check your blood glucose to get the most useful information. You may want to check before you eat breakfast and occasionally two hours after meals. People with type 2 diabetes who take insulin should check more often, and more specifics will be discussed in a later chapter on medications.

Most Common Times to Check

- Before breakfast
- Two hours after breakfast
- Before lunch
- Two hours after lunch
- Before dinner
- Two hours after dinner
- Before bedtime

Some people may want to do more focused testing to evaluate how a particular activity, like using a stair climber for 30 minutes, affects their blood glucose. Focused testing involves taking a blood glucose reading right before and after the activity.

More monitoring will give you more information about your blood glucose. However, if you have a limited amount of test strips under your health care insurance, you may want to talk with your health care provider about how to use your strips wisely.

Consider extra blood glucose checks if you:

- Feel stressed out
- Change exercise or diet
- Start a new medication that can affect your blood glucose
- Make changes in the dose of diabetes medication or insulin
- Suspect high or low blood glucose
- Have a cold or other sickness
- Are traveling and therefore outside of your normal routine
- Before and after exercise or during if it's more than an hour

HYPOGLYCEMIA

Abnormally low blood glucose is called hypoglycemia. It is usually defined as less than 70–80 mg/dl, but you and your health care provider should discuss this number. Low blood glucose can happen to anyone, although people taking insulin or other diabetes medications such as sulfonylureas are more susceptible. If unnoticed or untreated, hypoglycemia can make you feel or act out-of-sorts and even pass out. It can be dangerous to you and others especially when driving a vehicle. Hypoglycemia that isn't treated for a long time may cause seizure, coma, and even death.

Any number of situations can cause hypoglycemia. Perhaps you ate less at lunch than usual, ate lunch later, or skipped it entirely. Perhaps you have a cold or you drank too much wine on an empty stomach. Perhaps you exercised harder or longer than usual, without taking the extra exertion into account. Hypoglycemia is also common during sleep.

Checking your blood glucose is the only way to confirm hypoglycemia.

Many people experience warning signs of low blood glucose, but the warning signs are different for everyone. Most symptoms happen quickly. You'll want to learn your early signs of hypoglycemia so that you test and treat it right away. Explain common signs of low blood glucose to people close to you so that they can be on the watch for symptoms and have the tools to help you.

LONG-TERM HYPOGLYCEMIA

Scientists are studying the long-term effects of low blood glucose. One study has shown that severe low blood glucose was associated with a greater risk for dementia in older people with type 2 diabetes.

Warning Signs—Low Blood Glucose

- Anger, stubbornness, sadness
- Anxiety or nervousness
- Blurred or impaired vision
- Clamminess, chills, and sweating
- Clumsiness or lack of coordination
- Confusion
- Fast heartbeat
- Fatigue or weakness
- Headaches
- Hunger or nausea
- Impatience or irritability
- Lightheadedness or dizziness
- Nightmares or crying out in sleep
- Seizures
- Shakiness
- Sleepiness
- Tingling or numbness in lips or tongue
- Unconsciousness

Treating Hypoglycemia

Low blood glucose should be treated right away. An easy way to remember how to treat lows is the "Rule of 15" (see sidebar). You'll want to discuss with your health care provider whether the Rule of 15 is right for you, or whether you need to tweak it for your diabetes. Also, you can buy products—tablets, gels, and liquids—to specifically treat hypoglycemia. These fast-acting carbohydrates are easily counted for you in the container.

RULE OF 15

1. If blood glucose is below 70 mg/dL, eat or drink something with 15 grams of carbohydrate.
2. Wait 15 minutes.
3. Test again and if still below 70 mg/dL, eat or drink another 15 g carbohydrate.
4. Repeat until normal.
5. You may want to eat a snack if your planned meal is an hour or more away.

Sometimes, if you've had high blood glucose for a while and your blood glucose starts to come down, you may experience symptoms of hypoglycemia. However, you may not have low blood glucose at all. Talk to your health care provider about how to best manage this situation.

Glucagon

If hypoglycemia is not treated, you may become unconscious and unable to treat your own low blood glucose. For these emergencies, you'll need someone else to give you an injection of glucagon. Normally, glucagon is a hormone that your pancreas makes to raise blood glucose. Glucagon can also be manufactured as part of a portable kit that contains both a vial of powder and a syringe of liquid that are mixed before injection. Glucagon kits are available with a prescription and are recommended for anyone at risk for severe low blood glucose.

It is a good idea to teach family members or co-workers about how to use a glucagon kit and tell them to call 911 if symptoms don't improve or they don't feel comfortable giving an injection. You can download a free app from the company Lilly that tells you how to use a glucagon kit.

EXAMPLES OF 15 GRAMS OF CARBS

- Glucose tablets, follow package instructions
- Glucose gels, follow package instructions
- 4 oz fruit juice or soda (not diet)
- 2 tbsp raisins

HYPOGLYCEMIA UNAWARENESS

Some people with diabetes can't recognize the symptoms of low blood glucose, which is called hypoglycemia unawareness. If you suspect hypoglycemia unawareness, talk to your health care provider.

HYPERGLYCEMIA

High blood glucose is one of the signs of diabetes. High blood glucose is called hyperglycemia, and having it for a long time can damage your eyes, heart, nerves, and blood vessels. Many things can cause high blood glucose: perhaps you ate more than usual at dinner, forgot to take your medication, feel stressed or sick.

Some signs of hyperglycemia include: thirst; frequent urination; feeling "not right"; fatigue and lack of energy; dry and itchy skin; or blurry

DAWN PHENOMENON

Some people with diabetes have high blood glucose around 4 to 6 a.m.—called the dawn phenomenon. Your body naturally releases hormones that raise glucose at this time in the morning and you don't have the necessary insulin to counteract it. If you suspect dawn phenomenon, talk to your health care provider.

vision. The signs of high blood glucose may be harder to sense than low blood glucose. It is also possible to have mild hyperglycemia and experience no immediate symptoms. Still, there could be long-term damage.

Talk to your health care provider about how to detect and manage high blood glucose. For example, you may want to switch the dose or type of your medication, eat less or eat different foods, or exercise more.

Diabetic Ketoacidosis (DKA)

If left untreated, hyperglycemia can lead to diabetic ketoacidosis (DKA). People with type 1 diabetes are more likely to experience DKA than people with type 2 diabetes. DKA happens when blood glucose levels are consistently 250 mg/dL and above and tends to happen when people are sick or have missed their insulin. It is a dangerous situation that needs to be treated immediately.

During DKA, your body doesn't make enough insulin to get energy from the glucose in your blood. So instead, your body begins to break down fat to get energy from its cells. Together with a lack of insulin, the material coming from broken down-fat releases chemicals called ketones into your blood and urine, which can build up and become toxic. DKA can cause breathing problems, shock, seizures, coma, and even death.

You can test your urine for ketones using a simple test strip. Read the instructions on your ketone test strips: you'll either pee into a cup and dip the strip or hold the strip briefly in your stream as you pee. After you wait a specified amount of time, you'll compare the color of the strip to the included color chart to estimate the concentration of ketones in your urine. In addition, some blood glucose meters can measure the amount of ketones in your blood. You'll follow the meter's instructions, using separate ketone test strips and receiving a specific blood ketone reading on your meter.

Ask your health care provider in advance about when and how often to check for ketones. Some providers recommend checking when blood glucose is 240 mg/dL or above or every 4 to 6 hours when you're sick. Also, your health care provider will probably want you to call if you have ketones in your urine and may be able to give you instructions for treatment over the phone.

Warning Signs—Diabetic Ketoacidosis (DKA)

- Nausea
- Vomiting
- Blood glucose of 250 mg/dL or above
- Blurry vision
- Difficulty breathing
- Flushed sensation
- Weakness
- Drowsiness
- Intense thirst
- Dry mouth
- Need to urinate frequently
- Fruity odor on breath
- Lack of appetite
- Stomach pains

Hyperosmolar Hyperglycemic Syndrome (HHS)

Hyperosmolar hyperglycemic syndrome (HHS) is a life-threatening condition of high blood glucose and severe dehydration. It can happen to people with type 1 or type 2 diabetes, but it is most common in people with type 2 diabetes who *do not* take insulin, although anyone with type 2 diabetes can develop HHS.

Unlike DKA, which can come on suddenly, HHS develops over time and usually occurs because of something else like stress, infection, heart attack, or stroke. Not drinking enough fluids can also cause HHS—and can occur in elderly people who might be in a nursing home or hospital and don't have access to fluids or don't want to go to the bathroom.

During HHS, your body gets rid of extra glucose in your urine. Your urine becomes thicker and your body pulls fluids from other parts to thin it out. As a result, you have more urine and have to pee more frequently—sometimes leading to dehydration. If HHS continues, severe dehydration will cause seizures, coma, and eventually death.

HHS usually takes days or even several weeks to develop, which is why it's particularly important to drink lots of fluids when you're sick. For example, drink a glassful of fluid every hour and check your blood glucose more often. If you have a parent with diabetes in a nursing home, make sure water is always available and encourage him or her to drink water often. Also, some older people lose the ability to recognize their own thirst, so you may need to remind them to drink fluids regularly.

Warning Signs—HHS

- Blood glucose >350 mg/dL
- Dry, parched mouth
- Extreme thirst (although this may gradually disappear)
- Warm, dry skin, with no sweat
- High fever
- Sleepiness or confusion

SICK DAYS

It's easy for your blood glucose levels to be too high or too low when you're sick. You may not feel like eating, which can affect your blood glucose. Also, your body reacts to sickness by releasing certain hormones that raise blood glucose.

People with diabetes need a sick-day plan so that they know what to do ahead of time. Ask your health care provider to help you come up with strategies for managing your diabetes while you're sick. A sick-day plan may include: how often to check blood glucose, how to manage medications, what to eat and drink, when to call your health care provider, and what to tell him or her on the phone.

Even if you usually only check your blood glucose once a day normally, you'll probably want to check more often when you are sick. As a starting point, you may need to check your blood glucose every 3 to 4 hours, but ask your health care provider for more specifics.

Medication for Sick Days

If you take blood glucose medications, including insulin, it's important to continue taking them when you're sick. Remember, your blood glucose tends to go up when you are sick, even if you don't eat.

You may take cold medications or other medicine when you're sick. Some of the medicines, particularly cough and cold remedies, may have ingredients such as sugar or alcohol, which raise blood glucose. Read labels carefully for active and inactive ingredients. Look for sugar-free and alcohol-free versions of the same medicine. Ask your pharmacist or health care provider how a medication might affect your blood glucose.

For headache and fever, aspirin or Tylenol should be fine. People with kidney disease should avoid ibuprofen, the medicine in brands like Advil and Motrin.

Food and Drink during Sick Days

When you're sick, try to eat and drink the same kinds and amounts of carbohydrates as you normally would to keep your blood glucose on target. If you can't eat your usual foods, use your sick-day plan, which should include foods that are easy on your stomach and appealing to you, personally, when you're sick. You may want to set aside a small area of your cupboard for foods on your sick-day plan so you're prepared.

You may lose a lot of fluid if you experience a fever, vomiting, or diarrhea. Try to drink 3 to 6 ounces of fluids each hour by taking a few sips every few minutes. Non-diet soda or sports drinks with sugar and carbohydrates can help prevent low blood glucose.

PREGNANCY

Diabetes impacts many areas of your health, and it's true of pregnancy as well. Women with diabetes can have healthy pregnancies and healthy babies. It is even more important for women with diabetes to keep their blood glucose levels close to normal before and during pregnancy. High blood glucose puts your baby at higher risk for certain health problems: becoming very large; difficulty breathing; low blood glucose; jaundice (yellowing of skin), or injury to nerves of the arm during a difficult delivery. Although most of these conditions are treatable, preventing them in the first place is better for you and your baby.

Women with diabetes during pregnancy may have different medical histories coming into their pregnancies. There are several scenarios.

For example, a woman with type 2 diabetes may become pregnant. Or a woman may be diagnosed with diabetes for the first time when she visits a doctor early during pregnancy. Or a woman may find out she has gestational diabetes, a type of diabetes specifically identified during the second or third trimester of pregnancy.

Gestational Diabetes

All pregnant women without diabetes should now receive a test for gestational diabetes at 24 to 28 weeks. Although it's not something you planned for, diagnosing and managing high blood glucose is extremely beneficial to you and your baby. Lots of the time, changes to diet and exercise are enough to lower your blood glucose to a safe level. You'll work with your physician and perhaps a diabetes educator to come up with a diabetes care plan during pregnancy. In addition, make sure you're tested for diabetes 6 to 12 weeks after you give birth and every 3 years thereafter. Women with gestational diabetes have a lifelong risk of developing type 2 diabetes.

BLOOD GLUCOSE GOALS FOR WOMEN WITH GESTATIONAL DIABETES

- Before meal: 95 mg/dL or less
- One hour after meal: 140 mg/dL or less, or two hours after meal: 120 mg/dL or less

Planning for Pregnancy

If you already have diabetes, planning for pregnancy is one of the most important things that you can do for you and your baby. Talk to your health care team about the best way to prepare for having a baby.

Keep using birth control until your blood glucose levels are on target, as high glucose levels are linked to birth defects. Get into shape. Try to get fit *before* you become pregnant, to lose weight, improve endurance, strength, and flexibility and lower blood glucose. Make sure your health care provider checks for complications, particularly eye disease. Women with preexisting diabetes should have an eye exam during their first trimester and eye health should be followed closely throughout pregnancy, including one year after giving birth.

Care During Pregnancy

Once you become pregnant, you and your health care provider will come up with a personalized plan for managing your diabetes during pregnancy.

Exercise is important during pregnancy, although it's not the time to start a vigorous program. Instead, you will most likely be able to continue exercising like you were before pregnancy. If you were not exercising regularly, ask your physician about exercises that are safe for you and your baby.

Eating well is a basis for managing diabetes during pregnancy. Instead of cutting calories to lose weight, you need to eat foods to nourish your baby and help you avoid high and low blood glucose. The types and amounts of food may change throughout your pregnancy to keep up with your body's and baby's needs.

Some medications aren't safe to use during pregnancy, so you may switch to insulin. If you already take insulin, recognize that your insulin needs will probably change during pregnancy. Talk to your physician about any prescription or over-the-counter medications. In particular, be aware that many blood pressure and cholesterol medications are not recommended during pregnancy. As for all pregnant women, avoid alcohol, cigarettes, and other drugs because they may harm the developing baby.

If you can, plan to breastfeed your baby, which is good for your health and your baby's health. Breast milk provides essential nutrients and antibodies to your growing baby. And studies have shown breastfeeding lowers a baby's risk for obesity later in life.

BLOOD GLUCOSE GOALS FOR PREGNANT WOMEN WITH PREEXISTING TYPE 2 DIABETES

- Premeal, bedtime, and overnight glucose 60–99 mg/dL
- Peak post-meal glucose 100–129 mg/dL
- A1C <6

NEXT UP

Checking and managing blood glucose is just one part of your diabetes care plan. In the next chapter, find out how to eat well by choosing healthy foods.

Chapter 3

Food

Choosing healthy foods is essential to your diabetes care plan. The benefits are astounding. Eating well can help you lower your blood pressure, lower your cholesterol, meet blood glucose goals, and lose weight.

Unfortunately, misconceptions about diabetes and food abound. You may have heard that you can't eat certain foods if you have diabetes. Or you may have heard that you have to follow a specific diet. The truth is: there isn't a "perfect" meal plan for someone with diabetes.

Instead, choosing a variety of healthy foods—and eating them in moderation—is essential to eating well. You may enjoy salmon or grilled chicken, while someone else may be a vegetarian and prefer tofu. You may love to shop at the farmers' market or cook your own meals, while others may eat out at restaurants or need to take meals on the go.

In this next section, you'll find out about different types of foods, including the most nutritious, and strategies for incorporating them into balanced meals.

WHAT'S INSIDE:

- Types of Nutrients
- Drinks and Alcoholic Beverages
- Low-Calorie Sweeteners
- Vitamin and Mineral Supplements
- Balanced Meals: Carb Counting, Plate Method, and Low-Sodium Foods
- Food Labels
- Eating Out

TYPES OF NUTRIENTS

The three main types of nutrients in food are: carbohydrates, protein, and fats. Some foods contain an abundance of one type of nutrient while others may contain all three nutrients. You'll discover how each type of nutrient fuels your body and how to incorporate different types of nutrients into your meals in healthy ways. Also find tips about how to select a variety of foods and avoid unhealthy fare.

Carbohydrates

You'll find carbohydrates in starchy vegetables, starches such as bread and rice, dairy items, and fruit. It's a big group. Your body needs carbohydrates to provide energy for your body, and these carbohydrates often contain essential fiber, vitamins, and minerals.

Vegetables (the non-starchy kind) are full of vitamins, minerals, and fiber. And they don't include many calories or carbohydrates so you can eat these vegetables to your heart's content.

The fresh vegetable section of the grocery store is one of the best places to shop for vegetables because they are less likely to contain added ingredients like salt. Frozen and canned vegetables are also smart choices— just try to avoid ones with added salt or sauces. Many nutritionists recommend eating at least 3 to 5 servings of vegetables a day, but more servings are even better.

Common Vegetables (non-starchy)

- Artichokes
- Asparagus
- Bamboo shoots
- Beans (green, wax, Italian, yard-long)
- Bean sprouts
- Beets
- Broccoli
- Brussels sprouts
- Cabbage (green, bok choy, Chinese)
- Carrots
- Cauliflower
- Celery
- Chayote
- Cucumber
- Eggplant
- Greens (collard, kale, mustard, turnip)
- Hearts of palm
- Jicama
- Kohlrabi
- Leeks
- Mushrooms
- Okra
- Onions
- Pea pods and sugar snap peas
- Peppers
- Radishes
- Rutabaga
- Salad greens (chicory, endive, escarole, lettuce, romaine, spinach, arugula, radicchio, watercress)
- Sprouts
- Squash (cushaw, summer, crookneck, spaghetti, zucchini)
- Swiss Chard
- Tomato
- Turnips
- Water chestnuts

Courtesy: diabetes.org

Starches include grains like wheat and rice, but also starchy vegetables like potatoes, corn, dry beans, and peas. Starches also include grains in baked goods such as bread, pasta, pita bread, and tortillas, as well as recipes for hummus and soups.

The most nutritious type of grain is whole-grain, which means it contains the entire grain kernel (bran, germ, and endosperm). Whole grains have higher amounts of vitamins, minerals, and fiber than other refined grains such as white rice and white bread. And whole grains have been shown to lower your risk for cardiovascular disease.

To get all the benefits of whole grains, make sure the ingredients list says "whole-wheat flour," not just "wheat flour" or "enriched wheat flour." It should be the first ingredient listed. You can also look for whole-grain stamps on a package: the 100% whole-grain stamp means it contains at least 16 grams of whole grains or the basic whole-grain stamp means it contains at least 8 grams of whole grains.

Starchy vegetables and dried beans are also loaded with vitamins and minerals, and are low in fat and sodium. Fruits are packed with vitamins, minerals, and fiber. Just like vegetables, it's best to choose ones from the fresh fruit and vegetable section of the grocery store. Or choose canned or frozen fruit without added sugar, salt, or syrup.

15 Whole Grains

1. Bulgur (cracked wheat)
2. Whole wheat flour
3. Whole oats/oatmeal
4. Whole-grain corn/corn meal
5. Popcorn
6. Brown rice
7. Whole rye
8. Whole-grain barley
9. Whole farro
10. Wild rice
11. Buckwheat and buckwheat flour
12. Triticale
13. Millet
14. Quinoa
15. Sorghum

Courtesy: diabetes.org

7 Starchy Vegetables

1. Parsnip
2. Plantain
3. Potato
4. Pumpkin
5. Squash (acorn and butternut)
6. Green peas
7. Corn

Courtesy: diabetes.org

5 Dried Beans

1. Black, lima, garbanzo, and kidney beans
2. Lentils
3. Black-eyed and split peas
4. Fat-free refried beans
5. Vegetarian baked beans

Courtesy: diabetes.org

Common Fruits

- Apples (fresh or applesauce)
- Apricots
- Bananas
- Blackberries
- Blueberries
- Cherries
- Dates
- Figs
- Grapes
- Grapefruit
- Kiwi
- Mango
- Melon (cantaloupe, honeydew, watermelon)
- Nectarine
- Orange
- Papaya
- Peaches
- Pears
- Pineapple
- Plums
- Raspberries
- Strawberries
- Tangerines

Courtesy: diabetes.org

Protein

You can find protein in meat, dairy products, fish and shellfish, eggs, nuts, and legumes. Your body uses protein to help build tissues and muscles and to transport oxygen to cells through the bloodstream.

Meats such as pork, poultry, lamb, and beef can be good sources of protein, but try to choose lean versions that are lower in fat and cholesterol. Trim off excess fat and take the skin off chicken. How you cook meat makes a difference, too: grilling or cooking meat in a non-stick skillet is healthier than frying it in oil.

Dairy products such as milk, yogurt, and cheese are loaded with necessary protein and calcium. Consider low-fat versions of these dairy items—they still taste delicious.

Best Choices: Dairy Products

- Fat-free or 1% milk
- Plain non-fat or low-fat yogurt
- Unflavored fortified soy milk

Courtesy: diabetes.org

Fish, shellfish, and eggs are also excellent sources of protein. Fish and shellfish contain omega-3 fats, which have been shown to reduce cardiovascular disease, so try to eat two to three servings of fish a week.

Best Choices: Fish and Seafood

- Fish high in omega-3 fats: salmon, rainbow trout, albacore tuna, sardines, and mackerel
- Other fish: catfish, cod, flounder, haddock, halibut, orange roughy, and tilapia
- Shellfish: shrimp, scallops, clams, oysters, lobster, crab

Courtesy: diabetes.org

Legumes such as soybeans are an important part of vegetarian and non-vegetarian diets alike. They are chock full of protein and fiber. Don't forget nuts and seeds, which are super snacks, sides, or crunchy additions to salads. Dried beans such as black beans and kidney beans have starch, as mentioned above, and also protein.

Fats

Fat is the main nutrient in foods such as olive oil and butter. In many other foods, fats are found along with protein and carbohydrates. Our body needs fat to survive. In fact, it makes its own type of fat called cholesterol, which is used to make hormones and build cells. Other cholesterol comes from the food we eat—like fats. There are two main types of fat: healthy fats and unhealthy fats.

Healthy fats include both monounsaturated and polyunsaturated fats, which come from vegetables, nuts, and fish. They are considered healthy because they help lower cholesterol. Omega-3 fats found in fish, walnuts, and soybean products like tofu are also polyunsaturated fats.

GOOD AND BAD CHOLESTEROL

HDL (high-density lipoprotein) is often called "good" cholesterol because it helps take cholesterol out of the bloodstream and into the liver. LDL (low-density lipoprotein) is often called "bad" cholesterol because it builds up in arteries. In general, you want to raise HDL cholesterol and lower LDL cholesterol.

Monounsaturated Fats

- Avocado
- Canola oil
- Nuts like almonds, cashews, pecans, and peanuts
- Olive oil and olives
- Peanut butter and peanut oil
- Sesame seeds

Courtesy: diabetes.org

Polyunsaturated Fats

- Corn oil
- Cottonseed oil
- Safflower oil
- Soybean oil
- Sunflower oil
- Walnuts
- Pumpkin or sunflower seeds
- Soft (tub) margarine
- Mayonnaise
- Salad dressings

Courtesy: diabetes.org

5 Choices for Omega-3 Fats

- Fish: albacore tuna, herring, mackerel, rainbow trout, sardines, salmon
- Tofu and soybean products
- Walnuts
- Flaxseed and flaxseed oil
- Canola oil

Courtesy: diabetes.org

Saturated fats come from meat and dairy products and trans fats mostly come from the laboratory. Both fats can raise your cholesterol, potentially clogging your arteries and putting you at greater risk for cardiovascular disease.

The main sources of saturated fats are things like butter, whole milk, full-fat cheese, full-fat ice cream, and meat. Choose lean cuts of meat, use butter in moderation, and select dairy products that contain less saturated fat. Food labels now display the amount of saturated fat in grams and percentage per serving. In general, people with diabetes should aim for less than 10 percent of calories from saturated fat.

Trans fats are found in meat and dairy—but most are manufactured as food additives. Trans fats were originally developed by turning liquid fats into solid fats and added to products like cookies and crackers to extend their shelf life. More recently, we've discovered that trans fats are even worse than saturated fats, so you need to avoid them. Ingredient labels are required to display trans fats, which are often listed as "hydrogenated oil" or "partially hydrogenated oil."

Common Foods with Saturated Fat

- Lard
- High-fat meats: regular ground beef, bologna, hot dogs, sausage, bacon, and spareribs
- High-fat cuts of beef, pork, and lamb
- High-fat dairy: full-fat cheese, sour cream and ice cream, whole and 2% milk
- Butter
- Cream sauces
- Gravy made with meat drippings
- Chocolate
- Palm oil
- Coconut and coconut oil
- Chicken and turkey skin
- Fatback and salt pork

Courtesy: diabetes.org

Common Foods with Trans Fat

- Processed foods like snacks (crackers and chips) and some baked goods (muffins, cookies, and cakes)
- Stick margarine
- Shortening
- Some fast foods such as french fries

Courtesy: diabetes.org

DRINKS AND ALCOHOLIC BEVERAGES

Drinks are often forgotten when considering meals and healthy choices. Yet, drinks can be significant sources of calories and sugar that could increase your weight and raise your blood glucose.

Avoid sugary drinks such as soda, sugary fruit drinks, sweetened teas, and energy drinks. Water is always an option. Coffee, unsweetened tea, and diet soda are okay too. Choose low-fat milk, juices, or vegetable drinks with no sugar or sodium added—these drinks have calories, but they also have essential nutrients.

Drink alcohol in moderation. People with diabetes can follow the same recommendations as people without diabetes: women no more than one drink a day, men no more than two drinks a day. A drink is 12 ounces of beer, 5 ounces of wine, or 1.5 ounces distilled spirits such as vodka or whiskey. Don't drive or plan to drive if you've been drinking.

Alcohol can lower blood glucose, so you may want to eat something while you sip your beer or wine. Check your blood glucose before drinking to make sure your blood glucose isn't low. And you may want to check your blood glucose before you go to bed, as alcohol can lower blood glucose up to 12 hours after your last drink.

Certain diabetes medications that lower blood glucose could make you particularly sensitive to alcohol's effect on blood glucose. Talk to your health care provider if you drink regularly so that you can choose the best medication and strategies. Alcohol also contains calories. Some drinks such as beer, wine, and mixed cocktails contain carbohydrates, so you'll want to consider these drinks as part of your meal plan.

Tips to Cut Alcohol Calories

- Use no-calorie mixers such as diet soda, club soda, or water
- Put less liquor in your drink
- Choose light beer over regular beer
- Try a wine spritzer made with a small amount of wine and lots of club soda

LOW-CALORIE SWEETENERS

Low-calorie sweeteners are also called sugar substitutes and artificial sweeteners. They are much more powerfully sweet than sugar, so you need less to sweeten your food. They also contain fewer calories than sugar, so they can be alternatives for people with diabetes or people trying to lose weight. Five sweeteners have FDA approval (acesulfame potassium, aspartame, saccharin, sucralose, neotame) and another sweetener, called stevia, has been deemed generally safe by the FDA in moderate amounts.

Low-Calorie Sweeteners

Sweetener Name	Brand Names
Acesulfame Potassium	Sunett, Sweet One
Aspartame	Nutrasweet, Equal
Neotame	Neotame
Saccharin	Sweet'N Low, Sweet Twin, Sugar Twin
Sucralose	Splenda
Stevia	A Sweet Leaf, Sun Crystals, Steviva, Truvia, PureVia

Courtesy: diabetes.org

VITAMIN AND MINERAL SUPPLEMENTS

People with diabetes do not need to take vitamins or mineral supplements, unless recommended by their health care provider. For example, chromium, magnesium, vitamin D, and cinnamon are not recommended to improve blood glucose control. Taking n-3 fatty acids supplements such as DHA or EPA is also not recommended. Instead, try to get these important nutrients from the foods that you eat.

BALANCED MEALS: CARB COUNTING, PLATE METHOD, AND LOW-SODIUM FOODS

Now that you've heard about different types of foods—and some of the most nutritious—you'll want to try incorporating these foods into your meals.

Remember, there isn't a specific meal plan for people with diabetes. Instead, there are many food choices and meal strategies. Two of the most common are carbohydrate counting and the plate method. Choosing low-sodium foods may help reduce your blood pressure and risk of cardiovascular disease. Reading food labels and choosing healthy foods at restaurants are also important.

A diabetes educator and dietitian can help you come up with a plan for healthy eating. He or she is one of the most important members of your health care team. Both registered dietitian nutritionists (RDN) and diabetes nurse educators are trained to help you come up with food strategies to care for your diabetes. Your health insurance may cover sessions with a dietitian or diabetes educator, so read more about this in Chapter 7 on health care.

Carbohydrate Counting

Carbohydrates have the most impact on blood glucose after meals, so it makes sense that keeping track of carbohydrates can help you manage your blood glucose.

There isn't a "perfect" number of carbohydrates that people with diabetes should consume in a day. Instead, if carb counting sounds like an option, you'll work with your health care provider to come up your own optimal carb goals. Your goals might take into account the fact that you want to lose weight or you want to lower your blood glucose or increase your physical activity.

There are two types of carb counting: basic and advanced. In basic carb counting, the goal is to eat about the same amount of carbohydrate at about the same time each day. This helps keep blood glucose in your target range throughout the day. Instead of counting exact grams of carbohydrates in each food, you track the number of "carbohydrate servings" per day. On average, one serving of carbohydrate-containing food has about 15 grams of carbohydrate. In advanced carb counting, you track the exact number of grams in the food that you eat. You may have more flexibility to make changes from one meal to the next or to change your foods based on your medication or physical activity. For example, someone who uses insulin may need to count the exact number of carbohydrates in her breakfast so that she knows how much insulin to inject.

So how do you know the carb content of different foods? A food label is a good source of information, which lists the number of grams of carbohydrates per serving. Apps, websites, books, and handouts also list the grams of carbohydrates for foods. Your dietitian or diabetes educator can give you resources for counting carbs. Some restaurants now display the carbohydrate content of their meals on their website or menus.

Foods with About 15 Grams Carbohydrate

- Small piece of fresh fruit (4 oz)
- 1/2 cup canned or frozen fruit
- 1 slice of bread or 1 (6-inch) tortilla
- 1/2 cup oatmeal
- 1/3 cup of pasta or rice
- 4–6 crackers
- 1/2 cup ice cream
- 6 chicken nuggets
- 1 tablespoon syrup, jam, sugar, or honey
- 1 cup soup

Portion Control and Plate Method

It may sound basic, but portion management is a mainstay of managing your blood glucose. Eating appropriate portion sizes can help people with diabetes lose or maintain their weight.

The plate method, also called "Create a Plate," is a popular way to manage portions and choose healthy foods. It's a straightforward strategy in which you divide your plate into sections, filling each section with a different type of food.

For example, imagine you have a 9-inch dinner plate, and draw an imaginary line down the center making two equal sections. Next, divide one of the sections in half again. Now, you have two smaller sections and one large section of your plate. Fill the largest section with non-starchy vegetables like salad, green beans, broccoli, and carrots. Fill one of the small sections with a starch such as rice or potatoes and the other small section with a protein like chicken or fish. Drink a low-calorie

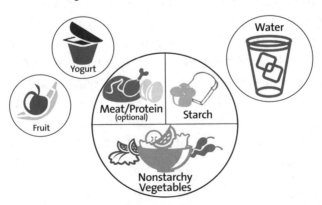

beverage like water and finish off your meal with a piece of fruit or dairy item like yogurt.

The advantage of the plate method is that you can use it at home and in restaurants—and you don't need any extra tools.

10 Tips to Eat Less

1. Serve food in the kitchen instead of at the table, so going for seconds is harder.
2. Eat slowly and stop when you just begin to feel full. Wait 10–15 minutes before getting seconds.
3. Savor your food. Don't watch TV or surf the web while you eat, so that you enjoy your food and notice when you're full.
4. Ask others to put leftovers away so you won't be tempted.
5. Don't go to the grocery store when you're hungry.
6. Write out a shopping list beforehand and buy only what's on the list.
7. Store food out of sight.
8. Eat a light snack before you go to a party so you'll be less likely to overeat.
9. Don't skip meals.
10. Don't forbid certain foods or you may want to eat them more. Instead, eat a smaller portion or eat fewer servings per week.

Low-Sodium Foods

Most people eat more sodium, or salt, than their bodies need, which can raise blood pressure and increase the risk for cardiovascular disease. When you have diabetes, high blood pressure also increases your risk for eye and kidney disease.

Many foods that don't taste salty still contain a lot of sodium. Cheese, salad dressing, deli meat, canned soup, tomato sauces, and many other foods all contain sodium. Even if you never put extra salt on your food, you could still be eating too much sodium.

The guidelines for sodium are the same for people with and without diabetes: 2,300 mg or less per day. Talk to your health care provider about your sodium goals and men-

ADA DAILY SODIUM RECOMMENDATION

Less than 2,300 mg per day

tion if you're considering using a salt substitute. Some salt substitutes can raise potassium, which is dangerous for people with kidney problems or who are taking certain medications.

Heart-Healthy Cooking Tips

- Use nonstick cookware so you don't need as much oil or butter.
- Cook food in 1 tbsp or less unsaturated oil, such as olive or canola oil.
- Use nonstick vegetable oil spray, wine, or low-fat broth instead of oils.
- Roast, grill, or broil meats on a rack so the fat drains off.
- Drain the fat as it cooks when pan-frying meat.
- Baste with broth or wine rather than pan drippings.
- Marinate meats and vegetables in lemon or lime juice, sherry, wine, vinegar, low-fat or non-fat broth, and fresh herbs for flavor.
- Microwave onions, garlic, peppers, and other vegetables in a bit of water instead of sautéing them in oil.
- Skim the fat from soups, stews, broths, gravies, and sauces. Chill them in the refrigerator so the fat is easier to remove after it floats and hardens at the top.

FOOD LABELS

Most packaged foods have "Nutrition Facts" printed on their label that include information like serving size, number of grams of various nutrients, % daily value, and the ingredients list.

Serving size information is found right under the "Nutrition Facts" label. It lists the serving size, which could be the whole box, half a box or just three pieces. All of the information listed on a food label is based on the serving size. So if the serving size of your cereal is 1/2 cup and contains 15 grams of carbohydrates and you eat 1 cup, then you're eating 30 grams of carbohydrates. The label also lists the number of servings per container.

The next section contains "Amount per Serving." It includes calories and calories from fat, which are important to consider if you're watching your weight. It also includes total fat, saturated fat, trans fat, cholesterol, sodium, total carbohydrate, and protein (in grams or milligrams).

You may want to pay particular attention to the total carbohydrates in a serving, as this number affects your blood glucose. The total fat is also important, as well as the saturated and trans fat. Lowering saturated and trans fats is important for people with diabetes. Also, check out the grams of sodium and remember that you're aiming for 2,300 mg or less a day.

Labels list the percent daily value of nutrients and are based on a 2,000-calorie diet. You don't need to know all the recommended daily values when you shop, and it may be easier to focus on the total amounts of nutrients per serving.

The ingredients section lists the main ingredient first and the rest of the ingredients in descending order. Keep your eye out for ingredients like whole grains listed first and avoid ingredients such as hydrogenated oil or partially hydrogenated oil.

Nutrition Facts

Serving Size 1 cup (53g/1.9 oz)
Servings Per Container About 8

Amount Per Serving

Calories 190	Calories from Fat 25

	% Daily Value**
Total Fat 3g*	5%
Saturated Fat 0g	0%
Trans Fat 0g	
Cholesterol 0mg	0%
Sodium 95mg	4%
Total Carbohydrate 36g	12%
Dietary Fiber 8g	32%
Sugars 13g	
Protein 9g	14%

Vitamin A 0%	•	Vitamin C 0%	
Calcium 4%	•	Iron 10%	

*Amount in Cereal. One half cup of fat free milk contributes an additional 40 calories, 65mg sodium, 6g total carbohydrates (6g sugars), and 4g protein.
**Percent Daily Values are based on a 2,000 calorie diet. Your Daily Values may be higher or lower depending on your calorie needs.

		Calories:	2,000	2,500
Total Fat	Less than		65g	80g
Sat Fat	Less than		20g	25g
Cholesterol	Less than		300mg	300mg
Sodium	Less than		2,400mg	2,400mg
Total Carbohydrate			300g	375g
Dietary Fiber			25g	30g

Calories per gram:
Fat 9 • Carbohydrate 4 • Protein 4

EATING OUT

Today, more and more restaurants are offering "lite" and "heart healthy" foods. You can usually find sugar substitutes, diet beverages, reduced-calorie salad dressings, low-fat milk, and salt substitutes. It's also easier to find salads, fish and seafood, vegetables, baked or broiled food, and whole-grain breads, rice, and pastas.

Many restaurants provide the nutritional value of meals such as the calories, carbohydrates, sodium, and fats. You can ask the chef to prepare a dish differently, such as by omitting ingredients like butter or broiling instead of frying food. Swapping vegetables for potatoes, rice, or pasta is another option.

If you take diabetes medication, you'll want to think about *when* you eat out as well. Eating at the expected time helps keep your blood glucose in your target range. If your meal is going to be later than usual, prepare by having a snack or adjusting your medications accordingly. If dinner will be very late, eat your bedtime snack before dinner.

11 Tips for Eating Out

1. Pick a restaurant that offers a variety of choices.
2. Ask the server about the size and ingredients of dishes.
3. Try to eat the same size servings that you eat at home.
4. Share with others if portions are large or ask for a doggie bag and put half of the meal in it before you start eating.
5. Eat slowly and take time to savor each bite.
6. Ask for broiled fish or meat to reduce fat.
7. Make substitutions or ask for a double portion of vegetables instead of french fries.
8. Ask for salad dressings, butter, or other sauces on the side.
9. Inquire about low-calorie foods, like salad dressing, even if they're not listed on the menu.
10. Substitute low-calorie or no-calorie drinks for alcoholic beverages.
11. Think creatively about the menu.

Fast Food

Today's fast-food restaurants are offering choices such as salads, grilled chicken, and wraps. However, there are still plenty of high-fat, high-carb, high-calorie choices out there. In fact, it's possible to eat an entire day's worth of fat, salt, carbohydrates, and calories in one super-sized meal.

PIZZA TIPS

Pizza can cause your blood glucose to go higher than expected and take longer to come down. Check your blood glucose at different times after eating pizza to learn how it affects you.

Keep these general rules in mind: Eat a variety of foods in moderate amounts, while limiting fat and sodium. Look at the menu carefully and choose wisely. Almost all fast-food restaurants provide the nutritional value of foods if you ask. If you have fast food for one meal, include low-fat foods and more fruits and vegetables in your other meals of the day.

Tips for Fast-Food Restaurants

- Breakfast: Try 1/2 a whole-grain bagel, toast, or english muffin. Order pancakes without butter and limit bacon and sausage.
- Load up on lettuce and vegetables with a salad. Go easy on the dressing, bacon bits, cheeses, croutons, and pasta salads. Try cottage cheese or salsa instead of dressing. Add garbanzo or kidney beans for added carbohydrate and protein.
- Order regular or junior-size sandwiches rather than super-sized or deluxe sandwiches.
- Skip the croissant and eat sandwiches on breads and wraps.
- Choose roasted, unbreaded, grilled, baked, or broiled fish and chicken.
- Stay away from double burgers or super hot dogs with extra cheese and sauces.
- Skip the cheese, which can add an extra 100 calories and extra fat and salt.
- Order items plain without toppings or rich sauces. Add lettuce, tomato, onion, and mustard instead.
- Dessert: Choose sugar-free, non-fat frozen yogurt or fresh fruit. Ices, sorbets, and sherbets have less fat and fewer calories than ice cream—but they can be high in sugar.

MEXICAN FOOD TIPS

Tacos, tostados, bean burritos, and other non-fried foods are healthier choices. Choose chicken over beef. Avoid beans refried in lard. Pile on extra lettuce, tomatoes, and salsa. Go easy on cheese, sour cream, and guacamole.

ASIAN CUISINE TIPS

Choose brown rice or whole-grain noodles, balanced with lots of vegetables including mushrooms, broccoli, cabbage, snap peas, bok choy, and more. Non-fried appetizers and dishes are healthier choices.

NEXT UP

Food is just one of the choices that you can make to live better with your diabetes. In the next chapter, discover how exercise, weight loss, quitting smoking, and staying up-to-date on immunizations can improve your health.

Chapter 4

Exercise, Weight Loss, and Other Healthy Choices

Exercising, losing weight, and quitting smoking are choices that you can make to improve your health. They are great choices for everyone—but particularly for people with diabetes.

Healthy lifestyle choices can help people with diabetes avoid or delay complications such as eye disease and stroke. More details about complications, and how to take care of your body and mind, will be covered in Chapter 6.

However, for now, keep in mind that a healthy lifestyle can give you more energy today and protect your body from harm down the road. Read on for ideas about making choices that fit your life.

WHAT'S INSIDE:

- Excrcisc
- Weight Loss
- Smoking Cessation
- Immunizations

EXERCISE

Exercise is one of the most positive choices you can make to help manage your diabetes. Exercise has so many benefits. You burn calories, which helps you lose weight or maintain your weight. Exercise improves your body's response to insulin, moves glucose out of the bloodstream, and reduces your risk of complications such as heart disease. It's a stress buster and mood booster to boot. And let's be honest, appearances make a difference. Exercise can help you look fit and feel better in your clothes.

SITTING IS BAD

Sitting for long periods of time (11 hours or more), regardless of your level of fitness, has been linked to a higher risk of death, according to a study of older women from the Women's Health Initiative.

Benefits of Exercise

- Lowers blood glucose and helps body use insulin better
- Lowers blood pressure and cholesterol
- Lowers risk of heart disease and stroke
- Burns calories to help you lose or maintain weight
- Increases energy for daily activities
- Helps you sleep better
- Relieves stress
- Strengthens your heart and improves blood circulation
- Strengthens muscles and bones
- Keeps joints flexible
- Improves balance to prevent falls
- Reduces symptoms of depression and can improve quality of life
- Prevents or delays onset of type 2 diabetes

It's never too late to start exercising or to exercise more. You can start exercising now even if you're overweight or you've never been physically active.

Getting Started Safely

To be safe, talk with your health care team before you start an exercise program. Your provider may need to check your heart, blood vessels, blood pressure, cholesterol, and A1C before you begin. Also, if you have complications of diabetes such as heart disease, high blood pressure, nerve damage, or kidney disease, ask about safe exercises for you. Moderate exercise, instead of strenuous activities, will probably be recommended.

If you're new to exercise, start slowly and be patient. Remember, your body is burning calories and working muscles whenever you move. Every little bit helps. So, incorporating physical activity is as much about changing habits as anything else. For example, take the stairs at work, join a community garden, or walk to the corner store instead of driving.

If you want to see how these changes add up, buy a pedometer and wear it all day. A pedometer is a small device that clips to your waistband or shoes and tracks how many steps you take during the day. Wear one for a few weeks, and record how many steps you take in a day. Try to add more steps each day or ask your health care provider about a recommended goal.

ACTIVITY TRACKERS

Activity trackers are newer, amped-up versions of pedometers. They count your steps, the number of miles you walk in a day, your heart rate, and even your sleep patterns. Some are clip-on and some are worn like watches—many sync to an app on your mobile phone to display results.

Types of Exercise

Once you get moving, you may want to add some more structured exercise. It could be walking in your neighborhood each day, taking an exercise class such as water aerobics, or joining a gym. Make sure you discuss your plan with your health care team to be sure it is safe for you. There are three basic types of exercise: aerobic, strength, and flexibility/balance. All three types of exercise are good for you.

Aerobic exercises are ones that make your heart beat faster and make you breathe harder. Walking, running, biking, and swimming are examples of aerobic exercise. Regular aerobic exercise can help burn extra glucose in your blood and improve the way your body uses insulin. It can also help you burn fat and shed pounds so that you reach your ideal weight.

Strength exercises—also called resistance training—are ones that work your muscles and make your bones sturdier. Using weight machines, free weights, or elastic bands are examples of strength exercises. Studies have shown that strength exercises lower A1C in older people with type 2 diabetes. And increasing muscle tone improves insulin sensitivity. Strong muscles and bones are less likely to become injured, too.

Flexibility and balance exercises help you stretch your muscles around your joints. Examples include yoga, pilates, and general stretching. When done correctly and safely, they can prevent injuries and falls. Keep in mind that everyone loses some flexibility as they get older, so doing flexibility exercises can help you stay more active and nimble.

Make sure that you're doing exercising correctly and safely so that you don't injure yourself. If you're trying new equipment in the gym, ask a trainer how to use it properly and how to adjust it. If you're taking a new class, tell the instructor that it's your first time and ask for advice. Don't be shy: there are no stupid questions.

Warm Up and Cool Down

Always try to warm up for 5 to 10 minutes before exercise and cool down for 5 to 10 minutes after exercise. A warm-up will slowly raise your heart rate, warm your muscles, and help prevent injuries. A cool-down will lower your heart rate and slow your breathing. Warm-ups and cool-downs can be as simple as doing your chosen activity, such as biking or walking, at a slower pace and with gentle stretches.

Start Slowly

Go slowly if you are just starting to exercise after a long time of little or no activity. Doing too much too fast can lead to injuries that could keep you from doing anything at all. Plus, it's easy to get discouraged and quit when you're sore and uncomfortable. Ease into physical activity to make sure you're being safe and keeping on track.

Try starting with just 5 minutes of aerobic exercise each day for 1 to 2 weeks. Then add 5 more minutes, and then another 5, gradually building up to 20 to 30 minutes of aerobic exercise several times a week.

If it seems like too much time to carve out at one time during the day, divide your exercise time throughout the day. For example, you might try brisk walking or stair climbing for 10 minutes at two different times in the day. You'll get the same benefits and you might find it easier to stick with shorter burst of activity.

Resistance training is often done in groups of repetitions, called sets. Some sets are multiple repetitions of light weights and other sets are fewer repetitions of heavier weights. It really depends on the type of strength exercise. Try to incorporate resistance training at least two times a week and allow your muscles to rest in between sessions.

Exercise Intensity

You can figure out how hard to exercise by measuring your heart rate. Ask your health care provider about your target heart rate and check your heart rate during physical activity to see if you're in range.

Measure your heart rate by taking your pulse. Place the tips of your first two fingers lightly over one of the blood vessels on your neck, just to the left or right of your Adam's apple (be careful not to check your pulse on both sides of your neck at the same time). Or try the pulse spot inside your wrist just below the base of your thumb. Count your pulse for 6 seconds and then add a 0 to the end. For example, if you counted 8 pulses in 6 seconds, then your beats per minute equal 80. You can compare your heart rate during exercise to your working heart rate to see if you're exercising at an ideal intensity. A heart rate device, worn as a chest strap or wristband, will automatically take readings and indicate whether you are exercising in your target range.

If you have nerve damage or take certain blood pressure drugs, your heart may beat more slowly and your heart rate would not be a good guide for exercise intensity. Instead, exercise at what you feel is a moderate level of exertion.

A good rule of thumb: You should be able to talk while you're exercising and you should not feel that you're exerting yourself too hard.

TIP TO GET MOVING

Park at the opposite end of the mall from the stores where you'll be shopping. Then, walk through the mall for extra exercise.

ADA RECOMMENDATIONS FOR PHYSICAL ACTIVITY

150 minutes a week of physical activity spread over at least 3 days with no more than 2 consecutive days without exercise. It is recommended that people with type 2 diabetes do resistance training at least twice a week.

CALCULATING YOUR TARGET HEART RATE

220 – your age = maximum heart rate in beats per minute.

Multiply your maximum heart rate times .60 for the lower end of range.

Multiply your maximum heart rate times .80 for the higher end of range.

For example, if you are 55 years old:

220 – 55 = 165 beats/min

165 x .60 = 99 beats/min

165 x .80 = 132 beats/min

Target Heart Rate= 99 to 132 beats/min

Exercise and Blood Glucose

Exercise can affect your blood glucose. Most of the time, exercise causes blood glucose to go down—a good thing for people with diabetes. If you take insulin or other medications, exercise can cause your blood glucose level to go too low. The opposite can happen during exercise, too: sometimes, your blood glucose rises when your body produces more glucose for muscles, but you haven't produced enough insulin.

The only way to know how exercise affects your body is to check your blood glucose before and after exercising. By monitoring your blood glucose, you'll begin to understand how your body reacts to exercise. After a few times, you'll have a better idea how exercise affects your blood glucose and you can make necessary changes to your medications, food, or exercise schedule. For example, you may need a pre-exercise snack. Talk to your health care provider about the best way to manage exercise if you have concerns.

Exercising when you're sick can make your blood glucose levels go down too low or up too high. If you exercise when you're sick, it may take longer for you to get better. You may have to ease back into your exercise routine after being sick. Ask your health care provider for advice about exercise and sickness.

Tips to Keep Motivated for Exercise

Convenience. Choose a type of exercise that you can do with a minimum of travel and preparation. Find something that you can fit into your daily routine, such as walking at lunchtime. Others may find that riding a stationary bike at home is more convenient.

Classes. Check out your community's exercise classes. Be cautious, as not all classes are of equal quality. Watch or try out a class before signing up. Make sure classes include a warm-up, heart-rate monitoring, and a cool-down with stretching.

Instructors. Look for instructors who are certified and have training in CPR. You might also want to ask whether the instructor has experience teaching people with diabetes.

Goals. Set realistic and measurable goals that allow you to track your progress. For example, if you're starting a walking program, walk for 10 minutes three times a week in the beginning. Then add more time and intensity.

Rewards. Reward yourself for following through on your exercise plans. If you planned to do strength training twice during the week and you did, do something special for yourself like buying new workout music. Try not to choose food as a reward.

Enjoyment. Find activities that you enjoy and partners who will help keep you motivated. You may like taking an exercise class for the social aspect or you may enjoy walking alone for the solitude and quiet.

Support. Asking a friend or relative to exercise with you can help you commit to a routine or just get out the door in the morning. Don't rely too heavily on a buddy if he or she has different goals or stops exercising.

Learning. Read up on activities that you enjoy by reading books, websites, or blogs online by fellow enthusiasts. You may be inspired—or learn a tip or two on techniques.

Cost. Check out classes or activities sponsored by your community or county government, which are usually more reasonable. Choose an activity that doesn't require specialized equipment, if you're concerned about cost. All you need to walk are comfortable clothes and a good pair of sneakers.

Novelty. Try something new if you're bored with the same old exercise routine.

DON'T FORGET WATER

Exercise makes you sweat, which means you're losing fluid. Drink liquids before and after exercise and during if the exercise is intense to replace fluids. Water is usually the best choice, so bring along a water bottle in a fun color or design that makes you want to take sips.

Times You Should NOT Exercise

- Dehydrated
- Short of breath
- Feel dizzy
- Ill or feel sick to your stomach
- Recovering from a serious injury
- Pain or tightness in your chest, neck, shoulder, or jaw
- Blurred vision, blind spots, or unstable eye disease

WEIGHT LOSS

Losing weight can be extremely beneficial for people with type 2 diabetes. It can help lower blood glucose. In fact, losing just 5 to 10 percent of your weight may be enough to lower blood glucose. Losing weight can also reduce the risk of complications and help you take a lower-dose medication. The benefits extend beyond your diabetes: weight loss can help you look better and feel better about yourself.

Always discuss your weight-loss plans with your health care team, as changes to diet and exercise can affect your blood glucose and medications.

To lose weight you must take in fewer calories than your body uses in a day. Most people lose weight by eating fewer calories or burning more calories—or both. Eating fewer calories means choosing smaller portions or selecting foods that have fewer calories (see previous Chapter 3 on food). Burning more calories means including more physical activity in your life or exercising more.

Eating less and exercising more may sound straightforward, but you'll probably want to take small steps to incorporate these goals into your daily routine. One of the key elements to losing weight is changing your behavior. And you may benefit greatly by working closely with a diabetes educator or nutritionist, who can help you come up with a plan to incorporate exercise into your daily life and create an action plan so you can achieve your goals.

Weight-Loss Programs

The number and variety of weight-loss programs is astounding: Weight Watchers, Jenny Craig, South Beach Diet, and the list goes on and on. Many diets are not geared towards people with diabetes, so you should always consult your health care provider before starting a weight-loss program. Your local hospital or medical center may offer weight-loss classes or support groups specifically for people with diabetes. Online physical activity and food trackers such as the ADA's MyFoodAdvisor may be helpful.

When evaluating a weight-loss program, consider one that helps you learn to replace old habits with new habits. A program that teaches you about nutrition and healthy food choices and encourages physical activity is ideal. Regular, follow-up visits to make adjustments and measure progress are also beneficial.

Bariatric Surgery

You've probably heard of bariatric surgery, or weight-loss surgery, which includes a group of procedures that change the body's digestive systems. The two main types of bariatric surgery are: gastric bypass surgery and lap-band surgery.

In gastric bypass surgery, a surgeon makes your stomach smaller, which makes you feel fuller and eat less food. The surgeon also disconnects your stomach from the first part of the small intestine and reattaches it to the second part of the small intestine, which means you digest fewer calories. In lap-band surgery, a surgeon places and tightens a band around your stomach to make it smaller, which makes you feel fuller and eat less.

Bariatric surgery can help obese people lose significant amounts of weight in the months and years following surgery. However, these are serious surgical procedures that carry risks. People with severe obesity (BMI greater than 35 kg/m^2) and type 2 diabetes may consider bariatric surgery, especially if they've had difficulty controlling their blood glucose or managing complications with medications or lifestyle changes.

Bariatric surgery can have a very positive effect on diabetes. In some cases, it reverses a person's diabetes. For example, studies have shown that bariatric surgery returned blood glucose to normal in 40 to 95 percent of patients with type 2 diabetes.

Many of these patients could stop taking blood glucose medications after surgery. The surgery's positive effect on diabetes appears to be independent of weight loss, although scientists don't know exactly how it works. More studies are needed on the long-term effects of bariatric surgery such as continued blood glucose improvement, sustained weight loss, and side effects.

SMOKING CESSATION

Smoking is dangerous for everyone, but especially for people with diabetes. Smoking puts you at risk for diseases of your blood vessels such as stroke, heart attack, and peripheral artery disease—and people with diabetes already have a higher risk of these diseases than other people. It increases your risk of all different types of cancer—not just lung cancer. And it can cause lung disease, such as emphysema and chronic bronchitis.

Some people can quit cold turkey. Many other people benefit from nicotine-replacement products and prescription medications. Replacement products include: patches, gum, lozenges, inhalers, and sprays. They work by putting a small amount of nicotine into your blood, which lets you gradually taper off your physical addiction. Some products can raise blood glucose, so always discuss your smoking cessation plans with your health care provider. Prescription medications, such as Zyban (buproprion), can also help people quit.

Support is a key to quitting smoking. Your company, health plan, or local hospital may sponsor a smoking cessation group. The American Lung Association offers group clinics and an online program to help people quit. The American Cancer Society has a program with telephone-based coaches and online tutorials.

4 Tips to Prepare to Quit Smoking

1. Set a quit date, and tell your friends and family. Make this a time when your life is fairly calm and stress levels are low.
2. Think of your reasons for quitting and write them down. Put the list where you'll see it every day.
3. Throw away your cigarettes, matches, lighters, and ashtrays.
4. Ask others for their help and understanding. Ask a friend who smokes to consider quitting with you.

Courtesy: diabetes.org

IMMUNIZATIONS

Make sure you're up-to-date on your vaccinations every year. People with diabetes and other chronic diseases may be more susceptible to the flu and pneumonia than other people.

Also, people with diabetes are twice as likely to become infected with hepatitis B than people without diabetes, according to the Centers for Disease Control. Hepatitis B can be spread through blood when people share diabetes care equipment like insulin pens and meters or in a hospital when patients accidentally share equipment. Vaccination is the best way to prevent hepatitis B.

Therefore, people with diabetes should have: annual influenza vaccine, pneumococcal vaccine, and hepatitis B vaccine for those aged 19 to 65 who have not yet been vaccinated. Don't forget vaccinations recommended for the general population such as the hepatitis B, pneumococcal, and the whooping cough and tetanus vaccine (Tdap).

Vaccinations

- Annual influenza "flu shot" vaccine
- Pneumococcal vaccine
- Hepatitis B vaccine

NEXT UP

Eating well, exercising more, and losing weight are some of the most important aspects of managing your diabetes. Medications also play a key role for many people. Medications include ones to manage your blood glucose, as well as ones to lower blood pressure and cholesterol. Read on for an overview of medications: how they work and what to consider when choosing a medications with your health care provider.

Chapter 5

Medications

Most people with diabetes take medications, such as pills or insulin, to manage their blood glucose. The good news is that there have never been more options available. It seems like every year brings new brands of medications and sometimes entirely new classes of medications to manage blood glucose.

Here, you'll find an overview of the most common diabetes medications: how they work, their benefits, and their adverse effects.

As a person with diabetes, you'll want to work with your health care provider to determine the best choice based on your lifestyle, health, and goals. There is no magic bullet medication for everyone with diabetes. In fact, you and your health care team may try different types and doses of medications to zero in on the best option. And your medications will most likely change over time as your body changes. This does not mean that you are worse or that you have not managed your diabetes well. It just means that your body needs more help.

Blood glucose medications are not the only drugs you need. Medications to manage your blood pressure and cholesterol can be just as important to your health. This chapter highlights the most common medications that people with diabetes take to keep their whole bodies running smoothly.

WHAT'S INSIDE:

- Blood Glucose Pills
- Blood Glucose Medications (Injected)
- Insulin
- Insulin Syringes and Pens and Inhaled Insulin
- Insulin Pumps
- Blood Pressure and Cholesterol Medications and Aspirin

BLOOD GLUCOSE PILLS

There are several classes of blood glucose pills approved in the United States, although some drugs are more favored than others. A class refers to how the medication works. Within a class, there are different types of medications and brands. For example, meglitinides are a class of blood glucose medications that include nateglinide (brand name Starlix) and repaglinide (brand name Prandin). Within each class, the safety and efficacy of a drug for a specific patient may vary.

In this chapter, you'll find the generic name for a medication in lowercase and the brand name in uppercase (sometimes in parentheses). You may hear older medications referred to by their generic name because they've been produced generically for a number of years. On the other hand, you may hear people refer to newer medications by their brand name because they are manufactured and marketed by a specific pharmaceutical company.

Classes of Blood Glucose Pills

- Biguanides
- Sulfonylureas
- Meglitinides
- Thiazolidinediones
- DPP-4 Inhibitors
- SGLT2 Inhibitors
- Other Drugs: Alpha-glucosidase Inhibitors, Bile Acid Sequestrants, and Dopamine Agonists
- Combination Pills

Biguanides

Biguanides include the most commonly prescribed medication for type 2 diabetes—metformin. It is often the *first* medication prescribed for people with type 2 diabetes, often at the time of diagnosis and sometimes if someone has prediabetes.

Metformin helps your liver release stored glucose more slowly. Metformin also makes your cells more sensitive to insulin so that they absorb more glucose. In turn, this lowers blood glucose. It doesn't help your body produce more insulin, like some other medications, so it's unlikely to cause episodes of low blood glucose. Metformin is a pill that is usually taken two times a day to lower blood glucose. It is also available in a liquid form.

Metformin was first approved in the United States in the 1990s under the brand name Glucophage and it is now available generically too. Glucophage XR is an extended-release version of the medication, which is now also available generically. Diarrhea, stomach discomfort, and nausea are the main side effects of metformin.

Sulfonylureas

Sulfonylureas are pills that help you make more insulin and lower blood glucose after meals. Most sulfonylureas are taken one or two times a day, before meals.

First approved in the 1950s, sulfonylureas now include a number of different pills: glimepiride (Amaryl), glipizide (Glucotrol, Glucotrol XL), glyburide (DiaBeta, Glynase PresTab, Micronase). They all improve insulin production, but they have different side effects and interactions with other drugs. They can cause low blood glucose, weight gain, upset stomach, and skin rashes.

Meglitinides

Meglitinides are pills that help you make more insulin and lower blood glucose after meals. They work quickly to stimulate insulin production after meals and they are eliminated from the bloodstream in 3 to 4 hours. Meglitinides are taken three times a day, just before meals.

Repaglinide (Prandin) and nateglinide (Starlix) are meglitinides that received FDA approval in 1997 and 2000, respectively. Side effects include low blood glucose, weight gain, upset stomach, back pain, or headache.

Thiazolidinediones

Thiazolidinediones, called TZDs for short, increase insulin sensitivity, which improves the way the body uses its own insulin and therefore lowers blood glucose. They are taken by mouth once or twice a day, with or without meals. They include rosiglitazone (Avandia) and pioglitazone (Actos).

TZDs first came to market in the late 1990s. In 2010, the FDA required Avandia to contain new prescribing information highlighting its increased risk of heart attack. However, in 2013, the FDA removed these prescribing restrictions. Pioglitazone (Actos) may increase the risk of bladder cancer and people with bladder cancer or a history of bladder cancer should not take this medication. Other side effects include an increased risk of bone fractures and excess water collection in body tissues in women taking Actos or Avandia. Combination pills that contain Actos or Avandia carry the same warnings.

DPP-4 Inhibitors

Dipeptidyl peptidase-4 inhibitors are pills that help lower blood glucose by helping your body make more insulin, keeping your liver from releasing stored glucose, and making your stomach feel fuller so that you eat less. You may sometimes hear DPP-4 inhibitors called "incretin-based" medications because of their role with incretin hormones.

INCRETIN

A type of hormone that causes an increase in the amount of insulin released from the pancreas after eating, even before blood glucose levels become elevated. Two medications, DPP-4 inhibitors and GLP-1 agonists, are based on the effects of these hormones.
Source: *The Diabetes Dictionary* 2nd Ed., American Diabetes Association

DPP-4 inhibitors are medications that inhibit or "block" an enzyme called DPP-4. It's helpful to "block" this enzyme because the enzyme destroys a hormone that can help lower blood glucose. In other words, the medication helps your body keep more of its blood glucose–lowering hormones around. DPP-4 inhibitors are taken by mouth once a day, with or without meals.

The first DPP-4 inhibitor, sitagliptin (Januvia), was approved in 2006, then saxagliptin (Onglyza) in 2009, linagliptin (Tradjenta) in 2011, and alogliptin (Nesina) in 2013. DPP-4 inhibitors all carry different side effects such as upper respiratory infections and headaches and different interactions with other drugs. The FDA is investigating rare cases of pancreatitis in people taking DPP-4 inhibitors and other incretin-based medications.

SGLT2 Inhibitors

Sodium-glucose transporter 2 inhibitors, also known as SGLT2 inhibitors, are pills that lower blood glucose by helping the kidneys remove excess glucose through urine. SGLT2 inhibitors block receptors in the kidneys that would normally reabsorb glucose into the bloodstream. Therefore your blood glucose is lower. They are taken once a day as a pill.

The FDA approved canagliflozin (Invokana) in 2013 and dapagliflozin (Farxiga) and empagliflozin (Jardiance) in 2014. SGLT2 inhibitors can lower blood pressure and improve weight loss. Possible side effects include urinary tract infections and dehydration. People with kidney disease or diabetic ketoacidosis should not use SGLT2 inhibitors and people with bladder cancer should not use Farxiga. The FDA also put out a warning that people on SGLT2 inhibitors may be at risk for developing diabetic ketoacidosis. So if you do not feel well, you should contact your health care provider.

Other Drugs: Alpha-glucosidase Inhibitors, Bile Acid Sequestrants, and Dopamine Agonists

Other drugs, such as alpha-glucosidase inhibitors, bile acid sequestrants, and dopamine agonists, may be used in specific patients, but are generally less favored because of efficacy, side effects, or how frequently you must take them.

Alpha-glucosidase inhibitors work a little differently than other medications. They are pills that you take at the beginning of meals to slow down how quickly your body breaks down carbohydrates and absorbs glucose. They can help flatten out the sharp rise in blood glucose that happens after you eat a meal. Acarbose (Precose) and miglitol (Glyset) are alpha-glucosidase inhibitors and they were both approved in the mid 1990s. Possible side effects are gas, bloating, and diarrhea.

Bile acid sequestrants are pills that were originally developed to lower cholesterol. In addition to lowering cholesterol, one bile acid sequestrant, called colesevelam (Welchol), has been shown to lower blood glucose, although scientists don't understand exactly why. Welchol is taken once or twice a day with a meal and drink or as a powder suspension. Side effects include upset stomach, constipation, interference with absorption of other medications, and nausea.

Dopamine agonists are medications that act like a chemical called dopamine in our brains. One dopamine receptor agonist called bromocriptine mesylate (Cycloset) is approved to lower blood glucose in people with type 2 diabetes. Unlike other blood glucose medications, Cycloset works primarily in the brain, although scientists don't understand exactly why it lowers blood glucose. Cycloset tablets are taken once a day within 2 hours of waking up and the dose varies from 2 to 6 tablets.

Side effects include low blood pressure, fainting, dizziness, upset stomach, fatigue, and low blood glucose. People with allergies to bromocriptine or who experience (fainting) migraines should not use Cycloset.

Combination Pills

Blood glucose pills also come as combinations of different medications
- glipizide and metformin
- glyburide with metformin (Glucovance)
- sitagliptin with metformin (Janumet and Janumet XR)
- linagliptin with metformin (Jentadueto)
- repaglinide with metformin (PrandiMet)
- saxagliptin with extended-release metformin (Kombiglyze XR)
- rosiglitazone with metformin (Avandamet)
- rosiglitazone with glimepiride (Avandaryl)
- pioglitazone and metformin (ActoPlus Met and ActoPlus Met XR)
- pioglitazone and glimepiride (Duetact)
- alogliptin and pioglitazone (Oseni)
- alogliptin and metformin (Kazano)
- sitagliptin and simvastatin (Juvisync)

BLOOD GLUCOSE MEDICATIONS (INJECTED)

People with type 2 diabetes can also use injected medications to help lower their blood glucose. Injected medications differ from pills in that they are injected under the skin rather than taken by mouth. However, keep in mind: they are not insulin. There are two classes of injectable blood glucose medications.

Injectable Blood Glucose Medications

- GLP-1 Agonists
- Amylin Analogs

GLP-1 Agonists

GLP-1 agonists help lower blood glucose by helping your body make more insulin, keeping your liver from releasing stored glucose, and making your stomach feel fuller so that you don't eat so much. GLP-1 agonists are "incretin-based" medications. However, GLP-1 agonists mimic a glucose-lowering hormone called GLP-1. In other words, the medication mimics the effects of a naturally occurring hormone that lowers blood glucose.

The first GLP-1 agonist, called exentide (Byetta), received FDA approval in 2005 and liraglutide (Victoza) in 2010. Byetta is injected before breakfast and dinner using a disposable pen with a 30-day supply of medication. Victoza is injected once a day. A once-weekly version of exentide called Bydureon was approved in 2012 and other once-weekly GLP-1 agonists called albiglutide (Tanzeum) and dulaglutide (Trulicity) were approved in 2014.

Side effects of all GLP-1 agonists include weight loss, nausea and vomiting, low blood glucose, kidney problems, potential for dehydration in case of vomiting, as well as inflammation of the pancreas. The FDA is investigating the increased risk of thyroid cancer in these medications, so you should not use them if you have a personal or family history of medullary thyroid cancer or an endocrine discorder called Men II.

Amylin Analogs

Amylin analogs help to lower the rise in blood glucose that can happen during and after meals. Amylin analogs act like a hormone in our body called amylin. Our pancreas releases amylin along with insulin when we eat meals to help lower blood glucose and make us feel full. Some people with type 2 diabetes don't produce enough insulin or enough amylin. Scientists can manufacture synthetic amylin in the laboratory, which can then be injected with a needle.

Pramlintide acetate (Symlin) received FDA approval in 2005 for people with type 1 and type 2 diabetes who use insulin. It is always used along with insulin to lower the spike in blood glucose that can happen after meals. You inject Symlin right before meals using a disposable pen. Side effects include episodes of low blood glucose and upset stomach.

INSULIN

Some people with type 2 diabetes need to take insulin because they don't make enough insulin or their body is resistant to insulin, or both. Whether or not you need insulin is highly individual. Some people need to start taking insulin immediately after they're diagnosed; some people take insulin years later; and some never take insulin at all. You should never think of insulin as a punishment or failure. It is really about what your body needs.

In the absence of diabetes, the body makes just one type of insulin— and it is released in both a steady, low stream throughout the day and night and in shorter, intense bursts when you eat food. Injected insulin comes in different forms to mimic the ebb and flow of insulin that naturally occurs inside our bodies.

The insulin you inject comes in different types, mixtures, and strengths. You'll read out about these differences below. How you *deliver* insulin also varies. You can use a needle, pen, pump, or inhaler to take insulin.

INSULIN ACTION

Type of Insulin	Onset	Peak	Duration	Names
Rapid-acting insulin	15 min	1 hr	2–4 hrs	insulin lispro (Humalog), insulin aspart (NovoLog), insulin glulisine (Apidra)
Regular or short-acting insulin	30–45 min	2–3 hrs	3–6 hrs	(Humulin R), (Novolin R)
Intermediate-acting insulin	2–4 hrs	4–12 hrs	12–18 hrs	NPH (Humulin N), (Novolin N)
Long-acting	1 hr	—	24 hrs	insulin glargine, (Lantus), insulin detemir (Levemir)

Insulin Types

There are four insulin types, distinguished by how they work inside the body. Each type of insulin has three different parts: onset (how quickly it starts working), peak (the time at which it works most effectively), and duration (how long it works). You'll find ranges for the onset, peak and duration of different types of insulin in the previous table. Insulin has ranges because it works a little differently for each person: it may work faster or slower for some or last longer or shorter periods of time for others.

Insulin Mixtures

Different types of insulin can be combined into mixtures to give the benefits of both. This type of insulin is called pre-mixed or mixed insulin. For example, an insulin mixture may combine intermediate-acting insulin with a smaller portion of short-acting insulin. The chart below includes information on the most common insulin mixtures.

HUMAN VERSUS ANALOG INSULIN

Human insulin is made in the laboratory by putting the human gene for insulin into bacteria, causing the bacteria to make human insulin. The insulin is then extracted and purified.

Analog insulin is engineered in the laboratory when scientists make changes to human insulin genes. The changes make analog insulin work more like the insulin inside your body, but with benefits such as different peak times and duration.

Insulin Strengths

The most common strength of insulin in the United States is U-100 insulin, which means it has 100 units of insulin per millimeter of fluid. U-500 insulin is also available for people who need a larger dose of insulin. U-40 insulin is still available in some parts of the world, but no longer in the United States.

INSULIN MIXTURES

70% NPH/30% regular	Humulin 70/30 and Novolin 70/30
50% lispro protamine/50% insulin lispro	Humalog Mix 50/50
75% lispro protamine/25% lispro	Humalog Mix 75/25
70% aspart protamine/30% aspart	NovoLog Mix 70/30

Insulin syringes sold in the U.S. are made for U-100 insulin.

Insulin Storage and Safety

Insulin comes in vials and these vials should be stored appropriately depending on when you use them. A vial of insulin that you are currently using can be left at room temperature for up to a month. Injecting insulin at room temperature is more comfortable than at colder temperatures. Unopened vials should be stored in the refrigerator. Do not put insulin in the freezer or allow it to warm in the sun or in a hot car because these extreme temperatures can destroy its potency.

Check the expiration date before opening an insulin vial. If the date has passed, don't use the insulin.

Look closely at the vial of insulin before you use it. Rapid-acting, regular, and long-acting insulin should be clear without floating pieces or color. Intermediate-acting insulin and insulin mixtures should be cloudy after rolling the bottle, but without floating pieces or crystals. If the insulin doesn't look right, return the unopened vial of insulin for an exchange or refund.

INSULIN SYRINGES AND PENS AND INHALED INSULIN

Most people use a syringe or a pen to inject insulin. With a syringe, you manually draw up insulin from a vial and inject it under your skin using the needle. With an insulin pen, you inject insulin from a pen that contains both a needle and insulin. Some people find insulin pens more convenient because they combine the needle and insulin in one device. Another option—inhaled insulin—has recently come back on the market.

Insulin Syringes

You may have to try several brands of syringes before you find one that suits you. Pick a syringe that is large enough to hold your entire dose for each injection. For example, if you take 45 units, you should not use a 30-unit syringe. Make sure that you can read the markings on the syringe clearly. Ask for the smallest and thinnest needles available for the size of your syringe or brand of pen.

Safely disposing of insulin syringes is important because they're considered medical waste. Used syringes have come into contact with human blood and the needles could accidentally hurt someone who is handling your trash. The best way to dispose of syringes and needles is to place them in a puncture-proof container with a tight-fitting lid before putting them in the garbage. Heavy-duty plastic or metal containers, such as a laundry detergent bottle, work just fine and you don't have to buy a special container. Remember to safely dispose of syringes when you're away from home or when traveling. You can buy containers for your home or for travel that are specifically made for syringe disposal.

Check with your local health department or waste disposal company to see if your community has special rules about disposal of syringes. The health department may be able to offer good advice.

Insulin Pens

Insulin pens come in two types: disposable and reusable. Disposable insulin pens come pre-loaded with insulin. They are thrown away when they're empty. Reusable insulin pens can be replaced with new, full insulin cartridges whenever they're empty.

Each pen holds a different type or types of insulin. And you select the dose of insulin by dialing a small knob on the pen. You'll also need to select a pen needle, which is screwed onto the insulin pen before you use it. Pen needles come in different lengths and thicknesses. Check with the manufacturer or consult the pen's directions about safe disposal of insulin pens.

Injecting Insulin

Insulin works best when it is injected into a layer of fat under the skin. Several areas of the body generally work well for insulin injection: abdomen, thighs, upper arms, and buttocks.

Your body absorbs insulin most quickly when you inject it into your abdomen. It's a good idea to inject insulin in the same area so that you know how quickly it will act each time. Or you may want to choose a different area of your body according to how fast or slow you want the insulin to start working. Either way, keep track of how your body responds by testing your blood glucose and recording the results.

Site rotation, or changing where you inject insulin, is also important to prevent skin and absorption problems. Hard lumps or deposits of fat can develop if you inject at the exact same place every time. So, you'll probably inject insulin in the same general area, but not the exact same place every day. It may help to think of each site as a circle on that area of your body. The circles, or injection sites, should be one inch apart. To rotate sites, use a different circle for each injection until all the circles have been used up. Then you start all over again.

The timing of your insulin injection also depends on the type of insulin you're using and when you're planning to eat. Ask your health care provider for the best advice about when and where to inject insulin.

5 Insulin Injection Tips

1. Inject insulin at room temperature. Using cold insulin right from the refrigerator can be more painful.
2. Relax your muscles in the area.
3. Puncture the skin quickly.
4. Keep the needle going in the same direction when you put it in and take it out.
5. Use sharp needles.

Injection Aids

Injecting insulin with a syringe takes some skill. And it can be difficult for people with poor eyesight or unsteady hands or a fear of needles. Injection aids can help people more easily inject insulin.

For example, people with poor vision can buy magnifiers that attach to a syringe to make the numbers more clear. People with dexterity problems can buy plastic or neoprene sleeves that fit over an insulin vial to make it easier to grip or caps that fit on top of a vial to prevent accidental needle pokes. You can even buy temporary tattoos that help you rotate your injection sites. New injection aids are always being invented, so check *Diabetes Forecast* magazine's annual Consumer Guide.

Inhaled Insulin

In 2014, the FDA approved the second inhaled insulin, called Afrezza, for people with type 1 or type 2 diabetes. Exubera, the first inhaled insulin, was taken off the market in 2007 due to poor sales. With Afrezza, you load a cartridge of insulin into an inhaler that you then use to breathe the insulin into your lungs. Typically, you take Afrezza, which is a rapid-acting insulin, just before meals. Side effects include sudden lung problems and people with asthma or chronic obstructive pulmonary disease (COPD) should not use Afrezza.

INSULIN PUMPS

Insulin pumps are small devices that deliver insulin directly through a needle or cannula inserted under the skin. A cannula is a thin, plastic tube, which stays put with a tiny adhesive patch. The insulin pump delivers rapid-acting insulin analog at a steady background stream, called the basal rate, throughout the day and in shorter bursts, called boluses, before meals. Some pumps require tubing to deliver the insulin from the device to the cannula in your skin. Some pumps don't have any tubing: the device has a needle you directly insert into your skin.

People choose insulin pumps because they allow greater flexibility about when and how to deliver insulin. You program the pump to tell it how much insulin you want and when you want it. Insulin pumps also come with a myriad of features such as data storage, remote controls, small increments of insulin, and wireless interaction with a blood glucose meter. You can always disconnect an insulin pump when you exercise or if you go swimming.

Onc insulin pump, called V-GO, is specifically designed for people with type 2 diabetes. It's a small, simple pump that attaches with a sticky patch and comes with a built-in needle for delivering insulin. It releases a continuous amount of background insulin; you can manually push a button to release insulin during mealtimes.

ARTIFICIAL PANCREAS

Manufacturers are developing devices that combine insulin pumps and continuous glucose monitors. The hope is that, someday, one device could both continually measure blood glucose and deliver insulin automatically much like a pancreas does inside our bodies. This technology is often referred to as an "artificial pancreas."

BLOOD PRESSURE AND CHOLESTEROL MEDICATIONS AND ASPIRIN

Besides medications to help lower blood glucose, many people with type 2 diabetes take medications to lower their risk of cardiovascular and other diseases.

Keeping blood pressure and cholesterol in the target range is essential for people with diabetes. Some people can achieve this through changes to diet and exercise. However, many people still need to take medications to maintain their blood pressure and cholesterol—and prevent damage to their heart, kidneys, and other parts of their bodies.

Blood Pressure Medications

Blood pressure is the force at which blood pushes through your blood vessels. It is given as two numbers, often as a ratio. For example, 140/80 or 140 over 80. The first number is systolic blood pressure: the pressure in your blood vessels when your heart beats and pushes blood out. The second number is diastolic blood pressure: the pressure in your blood vessels when your heart rests between beats.

People with diabetes are more likely to have high blood pressure, or hypertension, than people without diabetes. High blood pressure is commonly associated with heart attack or stroke. However, high blood pressure can also damage blood vessels throughout your body. It puts stress on your heart and brain—and also your kidneys and eyes.

Some people can lower their blood pressure by exercising, losing weight, and eating more healthy foods. Other people need to take medications, along with making healthy lifestyle choices, to lower their blood pressure. Many people with diabetes need to take two or more medications to keep their blood pressure in the target range.

ADA RECOMMENDATIONS FOR BLOOD PRESSURE

Blood Pressure <140/90 mmHg, with lower diastolic targets such as <80 mmHg for some patients.

Common medications used to treat blood pressure and protect the kidneys among people with diabetes are angiotensin-converting enzyme inhibitors (ACE inhibitors). ACE inhibitors include enalapril (Vascotec), lisinopril (Prinivil, Zestril), fosinopril, ramipril (Altace), and others.

Angiotension II receptor blockers (ARBs), beta blockers, and diuretics are also used to treat blood pressure. Blood pressure medications can have side effects and women who are pregnant should not use certain blood pressure drugs.

Cholesterol Medications

High triglycerides and low HDL cholesterol, called blood lipids, are more common in people with diabetes and can contribute to heart disease.

Some people are able to manage their blood lipids by eating healthy foods (with less saturated fat and cholesterol), exercising more, losing weight, and stopping smoking. Other people need to take medication, in addition to healthy lifestyle choices, to lower cholesterol.

You should receive a lipid profile, which includes your cholesterol and triglyceride levels, when you are first diagnosed with diabetes, at an initial medical evaluation or if you are 40 years old, and periodically thereafter.

Statins are the most common choice for treating cholesterol. Many people take statins without side effects; side effects are muscle and stomach pain.

LDL VS. HDL CHOLESTEROL

The dangerous type of cholesterol is called low density lipoprotein, LDL, cholesterol. You may have heard LDL cholesterol called "bad cholesterol" because it is the type of cholesterol that narrows or blocks your blood vessels the most. Blocked vessels can lead to a heart attack or stroke. Keeping LDL cholesterol low protects your heart.

The helpful type of cholesterol is called HDL cholesterol, which stands for high density lipoprotein. HDL is sometimes called "good cholesterol" because it helps remove deposits from the insides of your blood vessels and keeps your blood vessels from getting blocked.

Aspirin

You may also take low-dose aspirin (81 mg) to help lower your risk of heart disease and stroke. Most men over 50 years and women over 60 years with diabetes and risk for heart disease or stroke (such as a family history) take low-dose aspirin once a day.

NEXT UP

You've heard about a lot of different medications and technology. Remember, you'll work closely with your health care provider to make the best choices. Be sure to articulate your needs and preferences and tolerances. Look to have a conversation with your provider about the benefits and risks of taking a particular medication.

After all, you are the one taking the medication, so you are the most important part of the equation. Only you know how a medication regimen will fit into your life. Only you can feel the side effects of new medications on your body. And only you can articulate your preferences to your provider.

The last three chapters have outlined strategies for taking better care of yourself: healthy foods, exercise, weight loss, and medications. In the next chapter, you'll find more specifics about preventing damage to every inch of your body, from your brain to your toes.

Chapter 6

Body and Mind:
Prevent and Delay Complications

So far, you've learned about why it is important to manage your blood glucose and blood pressure. Now, you'll find out more specifics about *why* these efforts are so important to your health. The following chapter outlines how diabetes can affect different parts of your body such as your heart and skin and toes.

It's not news to you that people with diabetes have a greater risk of certain diseases—such as heart attack and stroke. However, taking care of your body can prevent and delay these complications. That is empowering information. In fact, studies have shown that patients and their providers have recently made great strides in reducing the rate of complications related to diabetes such as heart attack, stroke, kidney failure, amputation, and blindness.

This chapter targets the parts of your body most affected by diabetes: brain, eyes, mouth, heart, digestive system, kidneys, and nerves. You'll learn how to care for yourself with knowledge and skill. And don't forget your mood and sexual desire. Your sexual health and emotional health are essential to your mind and body. Read on for tips about how to keep your whole system running smoothly.

WHAT'S INSIDE:

- Brain
- Eyes
- Mouth
- Heart
- Digestive System
- Kidneys
- Legs and Feet
- Skin
- Sexual Health
- Emotional Health

BRAIN

Taking care of your blood vessels will help take care of that all-important organ: your brain. Blood vessels carry essential blood, oxygen, and nutrients to your brain. You can keep these blood vessels in good condition by keeping your blood glucose, blood pressure, and cholesterol on target. For almost everyone, this means eating healthy foods with less saturated fat and cholesterol. It also means losing weight, exercising, and stopping smoking. And it could also involve taking medications for blood glucose, blood pressure, or cholesterol—and possibly all three.

Blood vessels are the superhighways of your body, carrying blood rich in oxygen and nutrients. These super highways can become blocked with plaque and cholesterol, which leads to a condition called atherosclerosis or hardening of the arteries. Anyone can have atherosclerosis, but it is more common in people with diabetes.

When the blood vessels to your brain get blocked, parts of your brain can't get necessary oxygen and nutrients and these parts die. It's called a stroke. Sometimes it is also called a brain attack. There are different types of strokes, such as ischemic stroke, caused by a blocked blood vessel, and transient ischemic attack, caused by a briefly blocked vessel that eventually clears. Another type of stroke is a hemorrhagic stroke, which occurs when a blood vessel in your brain leaks or breaks. The most common cause of hemorrhagic strokes is high blood pressure.

A stroke can come on suddenly, so know the signs. Common signs of a stroke are difficulty walking or speaking; numb arms, legs or feet;

blurred vision; or headache. Immediately seek medical attention if you think you are having a stroke. The American Stroke Association calls these symptoms: FAST. *F* for face drooping, *A* for arm weakness, *S* for speech difficulty, *T* for time to call 911.

Treatments for blocked blood vessels to your brain include medications that prevent clots from forming or getting bigger or medication to lower blood pressure. Surgery can also remove a blocked blood vessel in your neck.

Tips for a Healthy Brain

- Lose weight to lower blood pressure, cholesterol, and blood glucose.
- Exercise to lower blood pressure, cholesterol, and blood glucose.
- Quit smoking to lower blood pressure and cholesterol.
- Take recommended medications for blood pressure, such as ACE inhibitors.
- Take recommended medications for cholesterol, such as statins.
- Keep your blood glucose on target with diet, exercise, and/or medications.
- Know the sudden signs of stroke. FAST. Face drooping, arm weakness, speech difficulty, time to call 911.

EYES

Your eyes also depend on blood vessels to keep them healthy. Over time, high blood glucose can weaken the blood vessels that lead to your eye so you want to keep your blood glucose under control to prevent damage. Studies have shown that lowering blood glucose can substantially improve eye health in people with diabetes.

Another way to protect your eyes is to get regular eye exams from an eye care specialist such as an optometrist or ophthalmologist. You should receive a dilated eye exam and a thorough check for any damage due to diabetes. Regular eye exams can detect damage that can be treated early to prevent eye diseases. Oftentimes, you won't notice any change in vision, so exams by an experienced eye specialist are essential to find any problems early when they can be more easily treated.

Three types of eye disease are more common in people with diabetes: retinopathy, cataracts, and glaucoma. Retinopathy is the most common and occurs when high blood glucose damages blood vessels to your eye. You can have nonproliferative and proliferative retinopathy.

Retinopathy

Nonproliferative retinopathy is common: one in every five people diagnosed with type 2 diabetes has it. In nonproliferative retinopathy, the small blood vessels in the retina bulge and form pouches called microaneurysms. The blood vessels weaken and leak some fluid, but it usually doesn't harm sight or get worse. If the disease progresses, the weak blood vessels leak a larger amount of fluid, along with blood and fats, causing the retina to swell. Usually the swelling won't impact your sight unless it occurs in the center of the retina (macula). The macula helps you see fine details. Swelling of the macula is called macula edema, which can blur, distort, reduce, or darken your sight.

Proliferative retinopathy is different and most people with type 2 diabetes do not go on to develop it. In proliferative retinopathy the damaged blood vessels completely close and new blood vessels grow in the retina and branch out to other parts of your eye. Sometimes, these changes affect your vision. Other times, the new blood vessels are fragile and rupture, causing problems.

Retinopathy can be treated successfully with laser surgery if it is found early. The laser patches up leaky vessels, destroys extra blood vessels, and discourages new ones from forming.

Cataracts

Cataracts are common in older people, whether they have diabetes or not. But cataracts can occur in younger ages in people with diabetes. In cataracts, your lens becomes cloudy, which affects your sight. The severity of a cataract depends on its size, thickness, and location on the lens. Cataracts can be treated with surgery in which the old, cloudy lens is replaced with a clear, plastic lens.

Glaucoma

Glaucoma is an increase in pressure in the eye that causes fluid to build up and damages the retina and optic nerve. It can lead to vision problems or vision loss. People with diabetes are 40 percent more likely to have glaucoma than people without diabetes. Glaucoma can be treated by reducing pressure in the eye using medication or surgery.

Tips for Healthy Eyes

- Keep your blood glucose on target with diet, exercise, and/or medications.
- Eat healthy foods, lose weight, exercise, and quit smoking to lower blood pressure.
- Get regular eye exams, preferably by an eye specialist familiar with diabetes.
- Pay attention to changes in your vision such as blurriness, dark shadows, difficulty seeing at night or while reading, or anything else unusual.

MOUTH

Your mouth is another important part of your body to take care of and keep clean. Mouths can be dirty places, as they're breeding grounds for bacteria and infections. Dental hygiene is important for everyone, especially people with diabetes. High blood glucose can hamper the body's own ability to fight infection and can support bacteria to grow in your mouth.

Keeping your blood glucose in the target range, cleaning your teeth well, and seeing a dentist twice a year will help keep your mouth healthy. You will also want to be on the lookout for signs of gum disease.

Cleaning your teeth involves both brushing and flossing regularly. Most dentists recommend brushing and flossing twice a day, but after every meal doesn't hurt either. Brushing removes surface food and plaque, a sticky form of bacteria. Flossing removes food and plaque from between your teeth. A soft toothbrush with rounded bristles is easiest on the gums. Be sure to replace your toothbrush every 3 to 4 months or sooner if the bristles are worn.

5 Toothbrush and Floss Tips

1. Place the toothbrush at a 45-degree angle to where your teeth meet your gums.
2. Gently move the brush back and forth in short strokes on your outer tooth surfaces.
3. Brush the inner tooth surfaces. Use the tip of the brush for the inner front surfaces. Brush chewing surfaces. Brush the upper surface of your tongue.
4. Use a good amount of floss: about 18 inches.
5. Gently guide the floss between your teeth until you reach resistance at your gum line. Hold floss against one tooth and gently scrape the side of the tooth, moving the floss away from the gum. Repeat with tooth on other side.

See a dentist at least every 6 months for cleaning to remove plaque and tartar (a hard buildup of plaque). Checkups are also good opportunities for your dentist to check for gum disease or other mouth infections. Dental x-rays can be used to check for bone loss and other problems.

Gum Disease

Gum disease starts when plaque forms on your teeth at your gum line. Brushing and flossing can remove plaque, but if it's not removed, plaque hardens into tartar. Plaque and tartar make your gums red, sore, swollen and bloody when you brush and floss—called gingivitis. Without treatment, gingivitis makes your gums pull away from your teeth, leading to pockets of bacteria and pus—called periodontitis. In this more serious situation, you may experience bone loss and need to see a periodontal specialist for treatment.

Tips for a Healthy Mouth

- Keep your blood glucose on target with diet, exercise, and/or medications.
- Brush and floss your teeth twice a day.
- Regularly look at your mouth for signs of infection, such as puffy, swollen gums.
- See a dentist twice a year for cleanings and necessary exams.
- Tell your dentist that you have diabetes.

HEART

Your heart is one of the most important parts of your body. Taking care of your heart means taking care of your blood vessels, which deliver blood and oxygen. You can keep your blood vessels clear and running smoothly by lowering your blood pressure, cholesterol, and blood glucose. A healthy diet, exercise, weight loss, smoking cessation, and recommended medications can help you achieve these goals.

Blocked or narrow blood vessels to your heart can cause a number of problems, such as chest pain (angina) or heart attack. People with diabetes are at higher risk: they are two to four times as likely to have heart disease or stroke than people without diabetes. Heart disease and stroke are both considered cardiovascular diseases. Cardiovascular diseases include problems in the heart or blood vessels, or both.

A common symptom of heart disease is angina, which is a pain or squeezing feeling in your chest. Angina is a sign that your heart muscle is working hard, but not getting enough blood for its effort. It can be relieved by medications such as beta-blockers, calcium-channel blockers, and vasodilators.

Heart attacks are another form of heart disease. A heart attack occurs when blood flow to part of the heart is blocked. Blood flow can be cut off by a buildup of fat and cholesterol in the blood vessels, called atherosclerosis. During a heart attack, part of the heart muscle dies or is damaged.

Signs of a heart attack include: chest pain or discomfort; pain or discomfort in your arms, back, jaw, neck or stomach; shortness of breath; sweating; indigestion or nausea; light-headedness; tiredness or fatigue. Yet, you may experience none or just some of the symptoms during a heart attack. Also, people with diabetes may have nerve damage that blocks the feeling of chest pain commonly associated with a heart attack. Call 911 immediately if you

WHAT'S THE DIFFERENCE BETWEEN HEART DISEASE AND CARDIOVASCULAR DISEASE?

Heart disease and cardiovascular disease are often used interchangeably. In other words, they mean the same thing. They both refer to diseases of the heart *and* its blood vessels, so they include things like heart attack and angina, but also stroke.

GOOD NEWS

A recent study showed that the rate of heart attacks has dropped more than 60 percent in people with diabetes. Strokes and amputations have dropped by 50 percent between 1990 and 2010. Kidney failure has dropped by 28 percent in people with diabetes. Scientists attribute these positive findings to improvements in self-care and improvements in how providers and health care systems manage diabetes. Lifestyle changes and medications to improve blood pressure, cholesterol, and blood glucose have also probably helped.

suspect a heart attack. Treatments for those who are at risk or who have had a heart attack include surgery to repair blocked arteries.

Tips for a Healthy Heart

- Eat healthy foods to lower blood pressure and cholesterol.
- Lose weight to lower blood pressure, cholesterol and blood glucose.
- Exercise to lower blood pressure, cholesterol, and blood glucose.
- Quit smoking to lower blood pressure and cholesterol.
- Take recommended medications for blood pressure such ACE inhibitors.
- Take recommended medications for cholesterol such as statins.
- Keep your blood glucose on target with diet, exercise, and/or medications.
- Know the sudden signs of heart attack: chest pain or discomfort; pain in other parts of the body such as back, arms, neck, jaw, or stomach; shortness of breath; lightheadedness or dizziness or cold sweat.

SLEEP APNEA

Sleep apnea, in which breathing stops and starts repeatedly during sleep, is more common in people with diabetes—particularly people who are overweight. It can cause disruptive sleep, make you sleepy, and increase your risk of cardiovascular disease. Talk to your health care provider if you or your partner suspect you might have sleep apnea.

DIGESTIVE SYSTEM

Your digestive system is another part of your body to focus on when you have diabetes. And your digestive system is partly controlled by nerves. It's easy to imagine the nerves to your fingertips or your little toes, which are called sensory nerves. Sensory nerves control our senses. It's harder to imagine the nerves that control involuntary movements such as digestion, which are called autonomic nerves. Autonomic nerves control involuntary or unconscious actions.

People with type 2 diabetes are more likely to have nerve damage, called neuropathy. High blood glucose can damage the structure of nerves and damage the blood vessels that carry oxygen and nutrients to nerves.

Specifically, this nerve damage can cause problems in the intestine, called gastroparesis. In gastroparesis, the stomach takes too long to empty because the signals to nerves and muscles are delayed. Gastroparesis can cause a number of problems such as heartburn, nausea, or lack of appetite. It can also interfere with your own good efforts to manage your blood glucose. For example, the delayed emptying of the stomach can lead to a spike in blood glucose after meals.

Keep your blood glucose on target to avoid damage to the nerves in your intestine and stomach. This will help your digestive system run smoothly. Talk to your health care provider if you are uncomfortable during or after eating, as this may be a sign of digestive problems.

KIDNEYS

Kidneys carry out the essential—yet unglamorous—job of filtering waste from your blood into your urine. They are the "cleaners" of our bodies. Your kidneys filter the blood that flows through the blood vessels in your kidneys. They retain what our bodies need and get rid of what we don't need through the urine.

Kidney disease, called nephropathy, is damage to the small blood vessels in the kidneys. Overworked, weak blood vessels may start to leak a protein called albumin. One job of albumin is to hold water in your blood so that it doesn't leak out of blood vessels. Leaked water can cause swelling in your ankles or feet or puffiness around your eyes. It can be one of the first physical signs of kidney problems.

People with diabetes are more likely to develop kidney disease if they have high blood pressure. It is the combination of high blood glucose and high blood pressure that can damage blood vessels in your kidneys. Early kidney damage can be treated by lowering blood pressure and blood glucose. So, focus on weight loss, exercise, quitting smoking, and reducing sodium to lower blood pressure. In addition, medications such as ACE inhibitors and ARBs can lower blood pressure. Try to keep blood glucose in your target range and take your blood glucose medications as prescribed.

Some people don't have any signs of early kidney problems, like swelling or puffiness. Therefore, it's important that your health care provider check your urine for albumin (a sign of kidney disease) using an albumin test. People with type 2 diabetes should have an albumin test every year. Another test of kidney function is called the estimated glomerular filtration rate (GFR). Eventually, if damage progresses and your kidneys start to leak waste into your blood, you may need dialysis to filter out wastes or a kidney transplant.

Tips for Healthy Kidneys

- Eat foods low in sodium to lower blood pressure.
- Lose weight, exercise, and quit smoking to lower blood pressure and blood glucose.
- Take recommended medications for blood pressure, such as ACE inhibitors or ARBs.
- Keep your blood glucose on target with diet, exercise, and/or medications.
- Look out for swelling in your legs or ankles or puffiness around eyes.
- Albumin test once a year to detect early problems.

LEGS AND FEET

Blood vessels from your heart extend all the way to the outer reaches of your body, including your legs and feet. So do your nerves. Damage to either your nerves or your blood vessels can affect your legs and feet. You'll want to keep your blood vessels healthy so that blood flows well to your legs and toes. Be on the lookout for symptoms and any sign of problems. Remember, the key to good foot care: inspect and protect your feet, and seek help early for any problems.

Your health care provider should give you an annual foot exam to make sure your feet are healthy. The exam should include tests to determine the sensation, blood flow, and bone structure of your feet. Take your shoes and socks off as soon as you get into the exam room of your health care provider. This will ensure that both you and your provider remember to check your feet.

Peripheral Artery Disease

Sometimes, blood vessels on the periphery (outer reaches) become clogged with cholesterol and plaque. It's called peripheral artery disease (PAD) and it's most common in legs. The buildup of plaque in blood vessels, called atherosclerosis, is similar to what can happen in your heart or brain. PAD can be painful, cause leg cramps, and make it difficult to walk. Decreased circulation to legs and feet can also make wounds much more difficult to heal or more likely to become infected. And PAD often goes undiagnosed because people mistake the pain and cramping for something else like arthritis or just getting old.

The good news is: your health care provider can easily test for PAD using the ankle-brachial index. The index measures the blood pressure in your arm compared to your ankle. And treatments for PAD usually involve lifestyle changes like exercise (often starting slowly to minimize pain), and smoking cessation.

Neuropathy

Nerve damage to the feet and legs, and sometimes the hands, is the most common form of neuropathy. People with this type of neuropathy may have numbness or loss of feeling; muscle weakness; tingling or prickling sensations; shooting or stabbing pain; pain on contact with bed sheets or clothing; the sensation of bugs crawling over the skin; or sensation of walking on a strange surface.

Another crucial thing to keep in mind with neuropathy is that you may *not* be able to feel pain. You may be less able to feel pain, heat, or cold in your feet. So, you may not notice infections or other foot problems, which can lead to larger problems when left untreated. Regularly inspecting your feet is the key to keeping your feet healthy. To protect

CARPAL TUNNEL SYNDROME

People with diabetes have a higher risk for carpal tunnel syndrome, in which the median nerve of the forearm becomes compressed at the wrist. It is a type of compression neuropathy. Symptoms include numbness, swelling, or prickling in your fingers—with or without pain—when driving a car, working at a computer, or other situations. Tell your health care provider if you have these symptoms.

your feet while swimming or wading, wear footwear made for the water. Wear shoes when walking on hot pavement or sand.

Keeping your blood glucose in the target range can prevent neuropathy and ease symptoms. Treatments for neuropathy pain include antidepressant medications such as duloxetine (Cymbalta) and/or other medications such as pregabalin (Lyrica). Interestingly, you don't have to be depressed for an antidepressant to help with nerve pain. Topical creams such as capsaicin can also relieve pain. Keep in mind: sometimes symptoms can feel worse, even after treatment, before feeling better.

Nerve damage can also affect the nerves that help you sweat. As a result, your feet may become dry and scaly or your skin may peel and crack. Soaking your feet will also dry out your skin. Use lotion to keep your feet moisturized, but avoid putting lotion between your toes where the extra moisture can lead to infection.

Basics of Foot Care

Inspecting and protecting your feet will keep them healthy. Below, you'll find out about common foot problems—and tips for avoiding them. Also, keeping blood glucose in your target range will help your body use its natural defenses to fight infection. And because you are less likely to be dehydrated when your blood glucose is not too high, your skin will not be as dry.

Try to protect your feet from calluses—areas of thick skin that can develop after prolonged pressure or friction. A corn is a callus on a toe. Corns and calluses can develop on your feet when your body weight is borne unevenly or when your shoes rub or are too tight. To prevent calluses, wear shoes that fit well. Buy comfortable shoes that leave room for you to move your toes. Wear shoes with low heels, so your weight is distributed more evenly, and thick soles that cushion and protect feet.

Padded socks can reduce pressure and friction and shoe inserts can better distribute your weight. Don't trim or cut a callus yourself because it could lead to infection. Also, never use sharp objects on your feet. Instead, see your health care provider if you develop a callus so that it can be removed properly and not lead to infection.

Protect your feet from ulcers, which are sores or holes in the skin. Untreated cuts, calluses, and blisters can cause ulcers, which commonly appear on the ball of your foot or bottom of your big toe. They can also develop on the sides of the foot from shoes that don't fit well. You may not feel an ulcer because of nerve damage in your feet. Therefore, it is important to regularly inspect your toes for signs of infection. See your health care provider right away if you suspect an ulcer on your foot.

Prevent poor circulation in your feet by exercising and quitting smoking. Poor circulation can make your feet feel cold and look blue or swollen. Wear socks to bed at night to keep feet warm. Do not use hot water bottles, heating pads, or electric blankets because they may burn your feet without you noticing. Test bathwater first with your elbow or use a water thermometer to avoid burning your feet.

How to Care for Your Feet

- Check both your feet each day. Look all over them. Compare one foot to the other. Look for cuts, blisters, scratches, ingrown toenails, changes in color, changes in shape, punctures, or anything that wasn't there the day before.
- If your vision is impaired, have a friend or relative check your feet or use a mirror to see the bottoms of your feet.
- Keep your toenails trimmed. Follow the curve of your toe. See a podiatrist if you can't trim them yourself.
- Call your provider if you notice sores or any other foot problem that are not better with 2 days.

CHARCOT FOOT OR JOINT

Charcot foot, also called neuropathic arthropathy, usually starts with a loss of feeling or sudden swelling, redness, and warmth in your foot. You may notice that you can't get your shoe on. Call your doctor immediately and keep the weight off your foot if you notice these symptoms. Early treatment for Charcot foot is crucial because continued walking can permanently damage the bones in your arch and ankle.

Tips for Healthy Legs and Feet

- Get an annual foot exam to check for blood vessel, muscle, and nerve damage.
- Check your feet for calluses or infection every day.
- Wear comfortable shoes that fit well—with good soles and low heels.
- Wear socks that fit, without holes or bumpy areas.
- Check for pebbles or other objects before you put on your shoes.
- Eat healthy foods to lower blood pressure and cholesterol and prevent PAD.
- Exercise to lower blood pressure, cholesterol and blood glucose and promote circulation.
- Quit smoking to lower blood pressure and cholesterol, and promote circulation.
- Keep your blood glucose on target with diet, exercise, and/or medications to prevent skin infections.
- Talk to your health care provider if you suspect PAD.

SKIN

Your skin is the biggest organ in your body—and also one of the most important to care for if you have diabetes. You want to keep your skin clear of infections and prevent dry skin. Keeping blood glucose in your target range will help prevent both infection and dry, peeling skin. Also, people with diabetes sometimes pass more urine, which can lead to dry, itchy, dehydrated skin. A dermatologist can help with more serious skin problems, so ask for a referral from your health care provider.

High blood glucose can encourage bacterial and fungal infections on skin and make your body's defenses less effective. Common bacterial infections include styes (infected glands of the eyelid), boils (infected hair root or skin gland), or carbuncles (clusters of boils). Staphylococcal bacteria cause these red, painful, pus-filled bumps. Tell your health care provider if you suspect a bacterial infection. Common fungal infections include jock itch in men, vaginal infections in women, and athlete's foot in both men and women. Most fungal infections occur in warm, moist, dark places such as your groin or feet. Over-the-counter medications may work for a fungal infection, but consult your health care provider if it doesn't clear up.

Tips for Healthy Skin

- Clean your skin regularly with warm baths and showers (hot water can dry skin).
- Hydrate skin by using moisturizers and moisturizing soaps.
- Drink plenty of water.
- Use a humidifier during cold, dry winter months.
- Keep other parts of your skin dry such as between toes, under arms, and groin.
- Protect skin from the sun by using sunscreen (don't forget tops of feet) and wearing a hat.
- Treat minor skin problems with over-the-counter products, but consult your health care provider if the problems don't improve.

SEXUAL HEALTH

Your sexual health is also important to your mind and body. Protecting blood vessels and making sure your blood glucose is in your target range keeps your sexual parts in good shape. For example, nerve and blood vessel damage can make it difficult for men to get an erection. And women with nerve damage may have more difficulty with vaginal dryness and reaching orgasm. Or urinary tract or vaginal infections can interfere with comfort and sexual desire.

Prevention is the key to sexual health. There are treatments for sexual problems for both men and women. Men can use medications, vacuum pumps, sleeves, penile rings, penile injections, or implants for erectile dysfunction. Women can use over-the-counter lubricants for dryness and treat urinary or vaginal infections with medications.

Remember that one of the most important components of sexual health is desire. Sometimes lack of desire may reflect a hormonal deficiency. Problems with arousal

MENSTRUATION

Women with diabetes may have more difficulty managing their blood glucose during certain periods of their menstrual cycle. This is generally caused by normal fluctuations in estrogen and progesterone. Keep records of blood glucose during your cycle and discuss any concerns with your health care provider.

could also stem from the delicate balance between mind and body. Recognize that managing your diabetes, like any challenge in life, can affect how you *feel* about sex. If you have concerns or lack of desire, talk to your health care provider or consider seeing a specialist such as a psychiatrist or psychologist. Don't be shy.

Tips for Sexual Health

- Take care of blood vessels by lowering blood pressure and cholesterol, exercising, eating well, and not smoking.
- Keep blood glucose in your target range to prevent nerve and blood vessel damage that causes ED or vaginal dryness.
- Discuss treatment for vaginal and urinary tract infections with your health care provider.
- Talk to your doctor, nurse, or a specialist about difficulty with arousal or lack of interest in sex.

EMOTIONAL HEALTH

Your mind, your mood, your body, and your environment—all impact your emotional health. Is it any surprise, then, that people with diabetes need to pay particular attention to their emotional health? Being in tune with your emotions can help you take care of and feel better about yourself.

Emotional health is a broad category that includes conditions like depression and anxiety disorder, but perhaps more commonly the feelings of anger, frustration, and fear that go along with managing a chronic condition such as diabetes. It's called diabetes distress.

Diabetes Distress

Diabetes distress includes the unique and sometimes hidden feelings of worry, fear, and frustration that come with managing diabetes. Sometimes, people call it "diabetes burnout." It is very common. Eighteen to forty-five percent of people living with diabetes experience diabetes distress and the number could be even higher upon diagnosis.

Recognize that diabetes distress is common among people with diabetes. It's normal to feel overwhelmed by the self-care that goes along with diabetes: taking medications, eating healthy foods, monitoring blood glucose, and exercising regularly. It's also normal to feel fearful about complications that might arise, such as a heart attack or kidney problems. It's normal to feel anxiety about getting adequate care and being able to afford medications and equipment. And it's normal to feel frustrated by how other people may behave towards you or unfairly judge you because of your diabetes.

Scientists are beginning to study and classify diabetes distress as something distinct from depression or anxiety. And they do know that high levels of diabetes distress can negatively affect A1C, your confidence, and your ability to care for your diabetes and your quality of life.

Talk to your health care provider about feelings of diabetes distress. Admitting and talking through feelings can be therapeutic. Your provider should be able to offer suggestions about how to cope with diabetes distress or refer you to a specialist.

Depression

People with diabetes are more likely to experience depression than people without diabetes. You may feel alone or set apart from your friends and family because of the extra work you do to manage diabetes. Perhaps you are scared or sad when you find out about a complication. Maybe you're down because you're having lots of high blood glucose readings despite your best efforts. Although feeling down once and while is normal, feeling sad and hopeless for two weeks or more may be a sign of depression.

Depression can be caused by all sorts of things, such as physical illness or medications. Talk to your health care provider if you feel depressed so that you can eliminate things that might be contributing to your depression. Your provider may prescribe antidepressant medication and recommend that you see a mental health specialist such as a psychiatrist, psychologist, social worker, or counselor. Remember, depression is a common and treatable condition. The first step is talking to your doctor or nurse about your feelings.

Stress

Everyone has stress in his or her lives—it's unavoidable. Stress impacts our bodies and minds in all sorts of different ways. For people with diabetes, stress can be problematic because it raises blood glucose.

Also, stress can make it harder to stick to healthy routines like eating nutritious foods, exercising, and managing your blood glucose. Stress can interfere with your sleep too.

You can learn to manage stress in positive ways that include both short-term coping techniques and long-term relaxation strategies. If you feel stressed in the moment, you may want to take a deep breath or try progressive muscle relaxation (see below). At some point in the day, find time to relax and reflect on your experiences.

Understanding Stressors

- What causes you to feel stressed? Stressors are different for everyone. Something that makes you stressed may not stress someone else or vice versa. Make a list of the people or things that stress you.
- How do you react to stress? Pay attention to how you feel and react when you're stressed.
- How do you handle stress? How you perceive a situation determines how much stress you feel. Try to handle stress in a way that makes you feel in control—in the moment and afterwards.
- Some stressors are problems you can solve. Others, like diabetes, cannot be solved and must be coped with instead.

Progressive Muscle Relaxation

1. Close your eyes and breathe slowly and deeply.
2. You'll start with the muscles in your face, working your way down to your feet and toes.
3. Inhale. Raise your eyebrows. Tense them. Hold for a count of three. Relax your eyebrows. Exhale.
4. Inhale. Open your mouth and eyes wide. Then close your mouth and eyes tightly. Squeeze. Hold for a count of three. Relax your jaw. Exhale.
5. Inhale. Bite down on your teeth. Hold down for a count of three. Relax your jaw. Exhale.
6. Inhale. Pull your shoulders up. Hold for a count of three. Relax your shoulders. Exhale.
7. Inhale. Tense all the muscles in your arms. Hold for a count of three. Relax your arms. Exhale.

8. Inhale. Tense all the muscles in your chest and abdomen. Hold for a count of three. Relax your chest and abdomen. Exhale.
9. Inhale. Tense all the muscles in your legs. Hold for a count of three. Relax your legs. Exhale.
10. Inhale. Tense all the muscles in your feet. Curl your toes. Hold for a count of three. Relax your feet. Exhale.
11. Inhale. Exhale any tension that might be lingering in your body. Breathe in energy. Take several slow, deep breaths. Enjoy the relaxation.
12. Gradually open your eyes.

Tips for Managing Stress

- Take a deep breath and practice progressive muscle relaxation.
- Exercise to release endorphins and counteract stress hormones.
- Get a massage, but check if it is safe first with your health care provider.
- Talk to a therapist, particularly one familiar with diabetes or chronic medical conditions.
- Join a support group for people with diabetes, in-person or online.
- Sleep the recommended 7 to 9 hours a day.
- Get away on a mini-vacation or take a long weekend.
- Soak in a warm bath, and use a bath thermometer if you have trouble feeling hot or cold temperatures.
- Spend some quiet time each day in prayer, reflection, or meditation.

Learning to Assert Yourself

Some people find it difficult to talk about what they need. They may be embarrassed to have differences or have their needs conflict with those of the people around them. Some people simply find it difficult to call attention to themselves. Others fear the imagined consequences of speaking up for themselves.

Getting what you need to effectively manage your diabetes can be a challenge, especially when it comes to relationships, or in the workplace or in the health care provider's office. Being honest and direct about what you need may make it easier for you and those around you.

Tips to Assert Yourself

- Learn to say "no." A simple "No, thank you," says that you respect yourself enough to act in your own best interest. You also respect the other person enough to expect that he or she will understand.
- Be firm. Decide what you need and find the best way to achieve it. For example, don't risk low blood glucose by waiting to eat just because no one else is eating.
- Be considerate. Some people may be uncomfortable when you take a blood sample or inject insulin. Give your companions a choice about watching you do these tasks.
- Maintain self-respect. If you respect yourself, you will have less difficulty explaining your situation and asking for help when you need it.
- Be direct. Explain things simply to others. Ask for what you need.

Your Support Network

You don't have to face the emotions and stress of diabetes alone. Your family, friends, support groups, and health professionals can help.

Family

Tell family members that you have diabetes and share what you're learning about managing diabetes. You'll also want to tell your immediate family how to handle medical emergencies such as low blood glucose. You can give them books, such as this one, or magazines like *Diabetes Forecast* that explain diabetes. Invite them to attend a diabetes education class or support group meeting. Encourage them to check out helpful websites such as diabetes.org.

Your health care provider may have tips for talking about diabetes with your family. Or you may want to bring along a spouse or your adult children to your next doctor's visit.

Also, talk about your diabetes care plan with your family. Explain why each goal is important to your health. Offer specific ways they can offer help, support, and encouragement. Keep in mind, you may experience frustration with family members who are not always supportive. Be patient. Focus on the positive choices that you can make to take care of your mind and body.

Friends

Talking to your friends about diabetes can be beneficial to you both. It may help to talk about frustrations and good outcomes with those who know and love you best. And your friends may better understand your efforts and goals when you explain them in the context of diabetes. Just like your family, offer books, magazines, and websites as resources for learning about diabetes. Tell your friends outright about specific things that would be helpful and supportive.

Support Groups

Support groups may be one of the best ways to cope with stress and feel better. In a support group, you can talk about your own frustration and listen to other people's experiences. Ask your health care provider about recommendations for support groups in your area. If you feel more comfortable online, check out a message board or online community such as one sponsored by the American Diabetes Association (community.diabetes.org). There are support groups for almost anyone, including people with type 2 diabetes, parents of children with diabetes, and family members of people with diabetes.

Mental Health Professional

A mental health professional can help you explore your thoughts, feelings, worries, and concerns about living with diabetes and other issues in your life. Counseling with a mental health professional can help you deal with your emotions, discover new approaches to old problems, make changes in your behavior, and learn new ways of coping. Mental health professionals include: psychiatrists, psychologists, counselors, and social workers.

Individual, couple, family, or group counseling are options, depending on your needs. Finding a counselor that you like is highly individual. You may need to talk to a few counselors before you find one that you like and feel comfortable with.

Tips for Emotional Health

- Recognize that diabetes distress is common, and identify strategies to manage it.
- Talk to your provider or a mental health professional if you feel

depressed or extremely sad for more than 2 weeks.

- Manage stress in positive ways such as by taking a deep breath and taking time for yourself.
- Try to assert yourself in a positive, honest, and direct manner. Ask for what you need to help manage your diabetes.
- Develop a support network, which may include family, friends, a support group, or mental health professional.

NEXT UP

You've read about how to keep your body and mind in good shape: from your head to your toes. You, the person with diabetes, will be the one most responsible for many of the preventative strategies and healthy choices that keep your system running smoothly.

Your primary care provider and your health care team will also teach you how to manage your diabetes effectively, help you set goals, evaluate your health, and administer necessary tests. The next chapter dives into the specifics of your health care: how to choose a primary care physician and specialists, making the most of doctor's visits, and navigating the health care system with diabetes.

Chapter 7

Your Health Care

Health care is big topic for everyone in America these days. It is especially important for people with diabetes. After all, you must take care of your health every day.

You'll also work with a team of health professionals who can help you set goals, navigate treatments, and evaluate successes and complications. In this chapter, find tips on how to choose your health care team—from your diabetes care provider to specialists such as dietitians and eye doctors. Learn how to make the most of visits with your health care team and how to get started with a diabetes education class.

Today, people are also learning to navigate new systems of health insurance coverage—from their jobs, from Medicare and other government-run programs, and from state-run marketplaces.

Find out about how changes to health insurance—including Medicare and new rules under the Affordable Care Act—affect you and your diabetes care.

WHAT'S INSIDE:

- Health Care Team
- Health Targets and Tests
- Diabetes Education
- Health Care Appointments and Hospital Stays
- Home Health Care and Long-Term Care
- Health Insurance

HEALTH CARE TEAM

A health care team is a group of health care professionals who help you manage your diabetes. You are the most important member of your health care team. After all, only you can manage your blood glucose, stick with an exercise program, choose healthy foods, and take your medication as prescribed. You'll be the first one to notice successes or problems. Most likely, you'll be the first person to take action. All team members rely on you to tell them how your diabetes care plan is working and when you need their help.

Your health care team may include: a diabetes care provider such as an endocrinologist or primary care physician, certified diabetes educator (CDE) and/or dietitian, pharmacist, mental health professional, exercise physiologist, eye doctor, foot doctor, dentist, or others.

Diabetes Care Provider

Your diabetes care provider will offer you advice about how to treat your diabetes and refer you to specialists as needed. You'll want to choose someone who has experience working with people with diabetes.

A diabetes care provider is typically an endocrinologist, although it could also be an internist or general practitioner with experience in diabetes. An endocrinologist is a medical doctor who has special training and certification in treating diseases of the endocrine system, such as diabetes. Some rural areas of the country have fewer endocrinologists or people may have to drive long distances to see these specialists. In this case, a primary care provider may be the best choice.

If you are choosing a diabetes care provider for the first time or thinking about switching providers, you'll want to do some research. Ask any friends or relatives with diabetes about providers whom they know and trust. You could also ask your current providers, such as an obstetrician/gynecologist or family practitioner, for a recommendation. Your hospital or a professional medical society should also be able to help.

Consider scheduling an appointment to talk with a potential diabetes care provider. Most providers charge for this time, so be sure to ask about the "interview" fee. During the interview, take time to evaluate the office and the staff. Do you feel comfortable with the staff and provider? Do you feel like they listened to you? Could you see yourself working with the provider to set goals and troubleshoot problems? You may want to ask about the provider's education and continuing education, experience in treating people with diabetes, and what to expect during treatment.

10 Questions to Ask a Potential Provider

1. How many of your patients have diabetes?
2. Do you treat more people with type 1 or type 2 diabetes?
3. How many people with type 2 diabetes do you see a month?
4. Do you follow the American Diabetes Association or some other standards for treatment?

PATIENT-CENTERED MEDICAL HOMES AND ACCOUNTABLE CARE ORGANIZATIONS

Patient-centered medical homes and accountable care organizations are big buzzwords in health care. Both are systems for delivering health care that aim to improve treatment of patients and reduce costs.

Patient-Centered Medical Home: A model for health care delivery in which the primary care physician works closely with the patient to provide comprehensive, high-quality, safe, and coordinated care. Physicians may receive bonuses for improving primary care services. Also called Provider-Centered Medical Home. Care managers or care navigators may be on hand to help people manage chronic illnesses such as diabetes.

Accountable Care Organizations: Essentially, a group of doctors and hospitals that share the cost and delivery of health care to patients. Under the Affordable Care Act, Medicare and Medicaid encourage providers to be part of Accountable Care Organizations to lower costs and improve care.

5. Do you have a diabetes educator or dietitian in your office or do you refer one?
6. How often will regular visits be scheduled?
7. How long is an average appointment?
8. Who covers for you on your days off?
9. What would I do in an emergency?
10. Are you part of a Patient-Centered Medical Home or do you have care management services available?

Certified Diabetes Educator

A certified diabetes educator (CDE) is a health care provider specifically trained to teach people how to manage and cope with diabetes. Diabetes educators come from any number of backgrounds. For example, a diabetes educator could be a registered nurse, mental health professional, pharmacist, or physician. Typically, a diabetes educator works in an office or hospital that treats people with diabetes.

The role of a diabetes educator is to work with you, the patient, to make behavioral changes so that you can better manage your diabetes. A diabetes educator may also help you coordinate and communicate with your health care team. Contact the American Association of Diabetes Educators online or by phone to find an educator in your area.

A diabetes educator can educate you about lifestyle changes as part of diabetes self-management training. This type of diabetes education is often covered by insurance and Medicare. More about diabetes education and its coverage will be discussed later in this chapter.

Registered Dietitian Nutritionist

A registered dietitian nutritionist (RDN) is an expert in food and nutrition. Food is a key component of your diabetes care. A dietitian can work with you to create a personal meal plan based on your food preferences, weight, goals, lifestyle, and medications. Keep in mind that a certified diabetes educator may also be a dietitian, so you may not need to see a separate person.

Your diet is not static. So, your foods and meal choices change when your weight, lifestyle, or other goals change. A dietitian can help you adjust your meals and food choices to fit your changing life and goals.

Dietitians should be registered by the Academy of Nutrition and

Dietetics. Look for the initials RD, which stands for registered dietitian, or RDN, which stands for registered dietitian nutritionist. RD and RDN credentials have identical meanings. The Academy of Nutrition and Dietetics recently offered the new credential of RDN to reflect that registered dietitians are both dietitians and nutritionists. For example, people may call themselves nutritionists but they don't have the same credentials, hours of study, degree, and continuing education as registered dietitians.

You might see the initials LD after a dietitian's name, which stands for licensed dietitian. Many states require that dietitians have a license.

Medicare and most insurers will cover sessions with a dietitian, which are called nutrition therapy services or medical nutrition therapy services. Check with your health insurer to see about coverage under your plan.

Your diabetes care provider or local hospital may be able to recommend a dietitian. The Academy of Nutrition and Dietetics, eatright.org, can also refer you to a dietitian.

What a Dietitian Can Do for You

- Help you choose a meal strategy or approach that works for you
- Provide tips for using the meal strategy, such as carb counting
- Educate you about healthy food choices, such as reducing saturated fat and sodium
- Describe how different foods affect blood glucose
- Make a sick-day meal plan
- Teach you how to read food labels
- Educate you about how to choose wisely when grocery shopping or eating out
- Turn a high-fat or high-sugar recipe into a low-fat or low-sugar recipe
- Recommend cookbooks and food guides

Pharmacist

A pharmacist is trained in the chemistry of drugs and how drugs affect the body. A pharmacist has at least a bachelor of science in pharmacy degree (BScPharm) or a doctor of pharmacy degree (PharmD).

Your pharmacist can help you in several ways, including free counseling on medications. Consider using one pharmacy with a pharmacist or staff of pharmacists who will become familiar with all your medications. Ask your pharmacist to print out or email a list of your medications and doses so that you can carry it with you or have it on file at home. It might come in handy if you are admitted to the hospital or if you need it for a doctor's appointment.

8 Questions for Your Pharmacist

1. How often should I take this medication?
2. Should I take the medication with meals or on an empty stomach?
3. What are the side effects?
4. Should I avoid any foods?
5. What other medications, including nonprescription, may interact with this new drug?
6. When should I take a missed dose?
7. How should I store the medication?
8. Are there any special precautions?

Exercise Physiologist

An exercise physiologist is trained to develop an exercise program based on your medical needs. He or she can show you safe exercises based on any problems, such as a heart condition or foot disorder. An exercise physiologist may also give you tests to determine your fitness and strength. Always check with your diabetes care provider before starting an exercise program to make sure it is safe for you.

Look for an exercise physiologist with a master's or doctoral degree in exercise physiology or find a licensed health provider who has graduate training in exercise physiology. Certification from the American College of Sports Medicine is a good sign.

Fitness trainers and instructors are different than exercise physiologists, but they can also play an important role in your exercise routine. Fitness trainers might be employed by a gym or club, and may include yoga instructors, cross-fit trainers, and others. Usually, trainers aren't certified to advise on medical conditions. Instead, trainers offer exercise techniques, routines, and motivation for clients.

Eye Doctor

Your eye doctor is either an ophthalmologist or an optometrist. An ophthalmologist is a medical doctor (MD) who detects and treats eye diseases, prescribes medications, and performs eye surgery. An optometrist is not a medical doctor, but carries a degree in optometry (OD), and is trained to examine the eye for vision problems and to perform vision tests.

Your eye doctor will examine your eyes for any changes, determine what those changes mean, and discuss how to best treat your eyes. The ADA recommends that you have a dilated eye exam and visual eye exam every 1 to 2 years. If you're making a new appointment, make sure to tell the office that you have diabetes and would like a dilated eye exam. A dilated eye exam involves using eye drops to enlarge your pupils, which makes your eyes more sensitive to light. You may want to bring sunglasses with you or make plans for a designated driver after your appointment.

Foot Doctor

A podiatrist or foot doctor is trained to treat foot and lower-leg problems. Podiatrists have a doctor of podiatric medicine (DPM) degree from a college of podiatry and have done residency in podiatry.

People with diabetes are more likely to experience foot problems than people without diabetes, so a podiatrist can be an important member of your health care team. The ADA recommends that you have an annual comprehensive foot examination. People with foot problems should have their feet examined at every visit. If you or your provider find any problems with your feet or lower legs, you may want to see a podiatrist. To find a podiatrist, check with your diabetes care provider, area hospitals, or the American Podiatric Medical Association.

Dentist

At first, it may seem odd to think of your dentist as a member of your diabetes care team. However, dentists have the important role of helping you maintain a healthy mouth and strong teeth. High blood glucose increases your risk of gum disease and other mouth infections. You should have a dentist appointment and cleaning every six months—and make sure to mention that you have diabetes. You may need to see a periodontist if you have periodontal disease.

Mental Health Professional

Mental health professionals include social workers, psychologists, and psychiatrists. You'll want to find a professional who is trained to help you with the emotional side of diabetes, including diabetes distress, anxiety, and depression.

Social workers can help you and your family cope with the stress and anxieties related to diabetes. They can help you locate community and government resources to help with medical or financial needs. Look for a licensed clinical social worker (LCSW) with a master's degree in social work (MSW) and training in individual, group, and family therapy.

A clinical psychologist has a master's or doctoral degree in psychology and training in individual, group, or family psychotherapy.

A psychiatrist is a medical doctor who can provide counseling for the emotional problems and stresses of diabetes and can prescribe drugs to treat these problems.

Other Specialists

In addition to the above-mentioned specialists, you may see a cardiologist for heart conditions, nephrologist for kidney damage, or neurologist for nerve damage. Your diabetes care provider can refer you to these specialists if needed.

HEALTH TARGETS AND TESTS

Your health care team will monitor your health and help you evaluate whether your diabetes care plan is working. How often you need to see members of your health care team will depend on your health, your blood glucose goals, and any changes that need to be made to your diabetes care plan.

Most people with type 2 diabetes have at least two checkups a year to evaluate their diabetes. Checkups help you and your health care team detect problems as early as possible. During a physical exam, your health care provider will check: height, weight, and body mass index; blood pressure and pulse; hands and fingers; eyes; feet; mouth, teeth, and gums; skin; neck; nervous system; and heart.

BLOOD AND URINE TESTS FOR ADULTS WITH TYPE 2 DIABETES

Test	Target	How Often
A1C, a measure of your average blood glucose over the past 2–3 months	Less than 7%	Twice a year or every three months if you change treatments or you're not meeting blood glucose targets.
Blood Pressure	Less than or equal to 140/80 mmHg	Every visit to your provider.
Lipid Profile	Statin therapy based on age and risk factors	At time of first diagnosis, initial medical exam, or at age 40 years and periodically thereafter.

Other Common Tests for Adults with Type 2 Diabetes

- Nerve function test using vibrations or touch to screen for neuropathy (yearly).
- Dilated eye exam to screen for eye disease (yearly).
- Ankle-brachial index to screen for peripheral artery disease in people over 50 or younger people with risk factors.

DIABETES EDUCATION

A great way to get a solid foundation in diabetes care is to attend a diabetes education program. To learn about local programs contact the American Diabetes Association, American Association of Diabetes Educators, local hospitals, county or state department of health, or your diabetes care provider. You may have a variety of programs to choose from, so ask for further information before selecting a class.

Most insurance plans cover diabetes education classes. It is often called "diabetes self-management training." Medicare Part B covers 10 hours of diabetes education the first year after diagnosis, plus an additional 2 hours every year after. Medicare or other insurers may require that you have a doctor's orders and that the program meet certain requirements.

Both the American Diabetes Association and the American Association of Diabetes Educators recognize certain programs so contact either association to find out about classes in your area.

Many programs will advertise that they meet the National Standards for Diabetes Self-Management Education and Support. Classes that meet these standards have skilled and experienced health professionals as instructors.

Diabetes education focuses on seven self-care behaviors: healthy eating, being active, monitoring, taking medication, problem solving, healthy coping, and reducing risks.

HEALTH CARE APPOINTMENTS AND HOSPITAL STAYS

Ever feel like your doctor's visit was too short? Or perhaps you only remembered an important question on the car ride home? You'll want to prepare for appointments with your health care providers to make the most of your visits. Preparation will help you and your provider tackle the most pressing issues, as well as cover the basics.

A hospital stay will also go smoother if you prepare for surgery or keep your blood glucose in range in case you're unexpectedly admitted to the hospital. The following section provides tips for making the most of doctor's visits and hospital stays.

Tips for Health Care Appointments

Communication is one of the most important aspects of a health care appointment, whether you're meeting your diabetes care provider or your dentist. Communication takes work between a provider and patient. It can be particularly challenging when you're feeling nervous, worried, or under pressure. Try to prepare for your appointment by writing down any questions or concerns ahead of time. Bring the list with you.

If your diabetes care provider is also your primary care physician, you might consider making a separate appointment to specifically discuss diabetes. For example, you might be crunched for time if you're scheduled for an annual checkup, but also want to cover questions and concerns with your diabetes management.

How to Prepare for Appointments

- Decide what you want to accomplish ahead of time.
- Write down any questions so that you don't forget.
- Write down emotional concerns or problems you're experiencing.
- If you're visiting your diabetes care provider or CDE, have your blood glucose readings handy from a logbook or computer.
- Bring a list of your medications and the doses. Or put all the bottles in a bag and bring the bag with you.
- Bring any health documents, such as discharge forms from a recent hospital visit or blood work results.

10 Ways to Make the Most of Your Appointments

1. Tell your provider what you want to accomplish at the start of the appointment.
2. Show your provider your list of medications and provide health forms.
3. Ask specific questions from the list you made.
4. Bring up emotional or other concerns. Don't wait to be asked.
5. Ask for a different explanation if your provider says something that you don't understand or that is too technical.
6. Bring a notepad or take notes on your phone.
7. Write down new instructions and information and ask your provider to repeat anything that you didn't hear clearly.
8. Remind your provider of previous decisions, conversations, symptoms, or lab results. It's not fair to expect your provider to remember everything.
9. If your provider offers recommendations that you know you can't or won't follow, say something. There are always alternatives.
10. Consider bringing a spouse or loved one, as sometimes a second pair of ears will hear things differently.

Tips for Hospital Stays

At some point in your life, you may have to go the hospital. Your reason for going to the hospital might have nothing to do with your diabetes, but it is still important that the hospital staff knows that you have diabetes.

Managing diabetes in the hospital is different than at home. For example, if you're hospitalized, you may not be able to follow your regular meal schedule or eat your normal foods. You may not be able to regularly exercise or you may not get as much rest as usual. Medications and other treatments in the hospital can raise or lower your blood glucose. All this, plus the stress of being in the hospital, can make it hard to keep your blood glucose in range.

However, keeping blood glucose levels on target is especially important in the hospital. Research has shown that people with diabetes get better faster, have fewer complications, and spend fewer days in the hospital when blood glucose goals are met.

Beforehand, talk to your diabetes care provider about how to handle a planned or unplanned trip to the hospital. Perhaps your provider can recommend an area hospital with expertise in treating people with diabetes. You could also do some research on your own. The ADA issues clinical guidelines each year—called the Standards of Medical Care for Diabetes—which includes recommendations for caring for people with diabetes in the hospital. You could call local hospitals to see if they've adopted these latest ADA Standards of Medical Care for Diabetes.

You'll also want to consider where your diabetes care provider has hospital privileges and which hospitals are covered by your insurance. Find out the answers to these questions now, so that if you suddenly need to go to the emergency room, you'll know the best hospital.

Immediately inform the hospital of your diabetes when you arrive. Many hospitals have medical doctors, called hospitalists, whose primary focus is your care in the hospital. A hospitalist can help manage blood glucose and troubleshoot other diabetes-related issues during your stay.

Blood Glucose in the Hospital

In the hospital, the goal is to keep blood glucose in your target range. The hospital staff will test and monitor your blood glucose, in most cases, so you don't need to do your own finger stick checks.

Keeping blood glucose in your target range can be challenging due to fluctuations in mealtimes, new medications, and procedures. If you normally take diabetes pills, you may be asked to stop taking them because they can interfere with other medications or make it more difficult to manage quick changes in blood glucose. Instead, you may be given insulin to manage your blood glucose while in the hospital. In most cases, you'll be able to return to your normal blood glucose medications when you go home.

Tips for Hospital Stays

- Tell the staff that you have diabetes.
- List all the medications you're taking: when you take them and the doses.
- Alert them to allergies, including medications or foods that may cause allergies.
- Tell the staff about any other medical conditions, such as high blood pressure, kidney disease, or eye problems.
- Describe any frequent low blood glucose reactions.
- Explain your meal strategies and diet, including special needs or allergies.
- If the hospital has a dietitian, request to speak with him or her.

Surgery

Your first question when considering surgery is whether it is necessary. If you have any doubts or just want reassurance, there is nothing wrong with getting a second opinion.

Second opinions can prevent unnecessary operations or help you consider alternative treatments. And they can put your mind at ease. Ask a health care provider you trust for a recommendation on a doctor who could provide a second opinion. Try calling the appropriate department of a major medical center or teaching hospital and ask for the name of a specialist in the field.

Reasons to Seek a Second Opinion

- A provider recommends surgery, long-term medications, or other serious treatments.
- You have doubts about the recommendation or just want reassurance from another provider.
- Your health insurance insists on a second opinion before paying full coverage.

If you decide to go ahead, talk to your diabetes care provider about how to prepare for an upcoming surgery. In general, you'll want to have your blood glucose within range before you enter the hospital. Research has shown that people with diabetes have better results after surgery when their blood glucose levels are on target and stable before, during, and after an operation.

Tell your surgeon and anesthesiologist that you have diabetes. Ideally, your diabetes care provider can work with your surgeon and anesthesiologist to come up with a plan for managing your blood glucose. Anesthesia and other drugs that you may take before, during, and after surgery can affect your blood glucose. Ask which medications you'll receive, how they affect blood glucose, and how your blood glucose will be managed.

12 Questions to Ask Before Surgery

1. Why do you suggest surgery for me?
2. What is the success rate of the surgery?
3. What does the surgery involve?
4. What are the risks and side effects of the surgery? And how likely are they to occur?
5. What will happen if I do not have the surgery?
6. Who will do the surgery?
7. How long will I be in the hospital?
8. How will my blood glucose be managed before, during and after surgery?
9. Will there be restrictions on my activities after surgery and for how long?
10. When can I go back to work?
11. Will I need follow-up care such as physical therapy or skilled nursing care?
12. What kind of rehab therapy should I expect?

Returning Home from the Hospital

Make sure you receive and understand your discharge instructions before you leave the hospital. Call your diabetes care provider when you get home to see if the plan you were given at discharge needs changes or modifications. Don't rely on the hospital to inform your doctor, in a timely manner, of your circumstances. Ask when you should come in for your next appointment with your provider.

HOME HEALTH CARE AND LONG-TERM CARE

In some cases, you may not be able to take care of yourself after surgery or a hospital visit. Sometimes this happens even if you originally planned to go home on your own, but your recovery is taking longer than expected. One option is to have a nurse or therapist come to your home as part of a home health care agency. Another option is an assisted-living facility, which provides help with daily activities. Still other options include skilled nursing facilities or nursing homes and rehabilitation hospitals.

Home Health Care

Home health care is a good option if you are housebound for a short time or you are bedridden with a long illness. Home health care agencies can provide: nursing care; physical, respiratory, occupational, or speech therapy; chemotherapy; dialysis; nutrition and diet therapy; and personal care such as bathing.

Home health care agencies may provide blood testing or bring a nurse into your home to administer drugs and other treatments. Home health care agencies include: the Visiting Nurses Association, the Veterans Administration, nonprofit public agencies run by city or county health departments, nonprofit private agencies, and for-profit agencies run by corporations. Ask for recommendations from friends or family, your diabetes care provider, local ADA affiliate, or local hospital.

10 Questions to Ask a Home Health Care Agency

1. How soon can services begin?
2. Are services available 7 days a week, 24 hours a day if needed?
3. Is there a minimum number of hours?
4. Will a detailed care plan be prepared before services begin?
5. Can I interview potential nurses or aides beforehand—is there a fee for this?
6. Can a request a change in a nurse or aide?
7. What are the fees for various services?
8. Will the agency submit bills directly to my health insurance?
9. Will I get a copy of these bills?
10. How often are bills sent?

Long-Term Care

You have several options if you need more care after your hospital stay including an assisted living facility, nursing facility, or rehab facility. Assisted living facilities offer help with activities of daily living like dressing, bathing, and getting around. Staff are on hand 24 hours a day, but they have little or no medical training. Residents often have private quarters and a lot of independence.

If you require more care, a skilled nursing facility or nursing home are options. Skilled nursing facilities can provide medical care (medication, rehabilitation), personal care (help with eating, bathing, and dressing), and residential services (room, food, social activities). Nurses and physicians are available 24 hours a day. Rehabilitation hospitals, sometimes called rehabilitation facilities, are specialty hospitals that provide rehabilitation for patients after surgery or serious illness.

Ask for recommendations about facilities from family and friends, your diabetes care provider, local ADA affiliate, or local hospital. Once you have found several good options, call and ask them to send you an information packet. Schedule a visit to the facilities and take along a family member or friend: the more eyes the better.

HEALTH INSURANCE

Health insurance has changed dramatically over the past few years, particularly for people with diabetes. It's essential that people with diabetes have access to health insurance so that they can afford medical care and treatments. People with diabetes also need insurance to help pay for medications and supplies, such as blood glucose meters and test strips.

Before, it was difficult for people with diabetes to get new insurance or change insurers: they were denied coverage or charged higher rates because they had diabetes. Now, under the Affordable Care Act, health insurers cannot discriminate based on pre-existing conditions. In addition, more options are available to consumers who are purchasing health insurance on their own through state or federally run health care insurance marketplaces.

In this section, you'll find an overview of different types of health insurance in the United States and specific coverage issues related to diabetes. The majority of Americans have health insurance through their employer or a government program such as Medicare or Medicaid. Keep in mind, the health insurance landscape is changing all the time. Keep abreast of the latest information at healthcare.gov.

Job-Based Health Insurance

If you have a job, you may have access to health insurance through your employer. Your employer may offer the choice of several or just one health insurance plan, with coverage for you or your spouse and dependents. Your employer pays a premium for the insurance and you make a pre-tax contribution.

For people with diabetes, it's important to know that no insurers—including ones through job-based coverage—can deny coverage or charge higher premiums because of your diabetes. Other new protections include: coverage for young adults until the age of 26 under their parent's insurance, free preventive care, and no limit on the dollar amount of coverage for "essential health benefits."

> ### AFFORDABLE CARE ACT (ACA)
>
> A federal law to reform health care in America that was enacted in 2010 and rolled out in phases through 2014. Under the law, people with diabetes have new protections, including not being denied insurance or charged more for services because of a pre-existing condition such as diabetes. Other benefits include free preventative care and no lifetime or yearly limit on how much insurers will pay for "essential health benefits" such as chronic disease management and medications.

Your health insurance options and benefits may be different based on whether you work for a large company or a small company. No business—large or small—*has* to offer health insurance for its employees.

However, new requirements under the Affordable Care Act require that large employers with 50 or more full-time employees pay a fine if they do not offer coverage that is affordable and adequate. Small businesses with fewer than 50 employees do not have to make these payments; they can purchase insurance for their employees under the Small Business Health Options Program (SHOP).

You can always visit www.healthcare.gov or call 1-800-318-2596 if you have questions about coverage for your diabetes under the Affordable Care Act. If you have questions about job-based plans or laws about insurance coverage, you can contact your state's insurance department: www.naic.org/state_web_map.htm.

Affordable Care Act: New Protections for Job-Based Plans

- *Coverage for Young Adults:* Young adults can stay on their parent's insurance plan until age 26 as long as the policy covers dependents.
- *Free Preventative Care:* Most health plans are required to provide certain recommended health services aimed at preventing disease at no charge.
- *Essential Health Benefits:* A minimum set of "essential health benefits" like hospitalization, prescription drugs, preventative services, and chronic disease management must be covered by all new individual and small group plans as of 2014.
- *No Lifetime Dollar Limits on Coverage:* Health insurance plans cannot set a dollar limit on the amount the insurance company will spend on "essential health benefits" over the course of the time the person is enrolled in that plan.
- *Summary of Benefits and Coverage:* Individuals have the right to get a plain-language summary of a health plan's benefits to help them better understand the plan's coverage and compare plans. The summary should be provided when shopping for coverage, when there is a major change in benefits, or any time a person asks for it.

Source: diabetes.org

Losing Your Job-Based Insurance

You will probably lose your job-based insurance if you lose or retire from your job. However, there are several options available: COBRA insurance, purchasing your plan in a health insurance marketplace, or joining a spouse's or parent's job-based health insurance.

COBRA stands for Consolidated Omnibus Budget Reconciliation Act. The federal law lets some people keep their health insurance for a limited time after they've left their job. Private companies and state and local government offices participate in COBRA. You'll have to sign up for COBRA within a certain amount of time after you've left your job.

HEALTH INSURANCE MARKETPLACE

A resource where individuals, families, and small businesses can: learn about their health insurance options; compare health insurance plans based on costs, benefits, and other important features; choose a plan; and enroll in coverage.

The Marketplace also provides information on programs that help people with low to moderate income and resources to pay for coverage. This includes ways to save on the monthly premiums and out-of-pocket costs of coverage available through the Marketplace, and information about other programs, including Medicaid and the Children's Health Insurance Program (CHIP).

The Marketplace encourages competition among private health plans, and is accessible through websites, call centers, and in-person assistance. In some states, the Marketplace is run by the state. In others, it is run by the federal government. Visit healthcare.gov to find your health insurance marketplace.

Courtesy: healthcare.gov

You'll probably have to pay more for coverage than you did when your employer paid a portion of your premium.

Health insurance marketplaces, also called health insurance exchanges, are another option if you lose your job-based insurance. In the marketplace, you can purchase your own individual plan. Normally, there is a specific enrollment period during which you must sign up for health insurance. However, losing your job or having your COBRA end qualifies you to purchase health insurance in a marketplace outside the typical enrollment period. Find out more about health insurance marketplaces above.

If you've lost your job-based insurance, you may also qualify to be added to your spouse's or a parent's plan (usually within 30 days of losing your own health insurance).

Medicare

Medicare is the federal health insurance program for people age 65 and older, people who cannot work because of certain disabilities, and people with end-stage renal disease. It is run by the Centers for Medicare and Medicaid Services, an agency of the United States Department of Health and Human Services.

Medicare covers hospital stays, health care provider visits, prescription drugs, and supplies like test strips. There are several parts to Medicare: Parts A, B, C, D, and Medigap. Each part pays for different types of health care. Parts A and B are what some people refer to as "original Medicare." Parts C and D have been added in recent years to provide more benefit options and prescription drug coverage.

Everything is not paid for under Medicare—and you may be responsible for certain co-pays and costs. Some people have secondary or "retiree" health plans that pay whatever Medicare won't cover. The publication "Medicare's Coverage of Supplies and Services" is a great resource and available for download at medicare.gov.

Medicare Part A

Medicare Part A covers *hospital* costs. For example, Medicare pays for medically necessary hospital visits, skilled nursing facilities, hospice, and home health care. If you're enrolled in Medicare, you don't pay a premium for Part A. This is because you paid Medicare taxes while you were working. However, you could pay a deductible for certain procedures.

Medicare Part B

Medicare Part B covers *medical* costs. For example, Medicare pays for visits to your health care provider, ambulance services, diagnostic tests, outpatient hospital visits, outpatient physical therapy and speech therapy, and medical equipment and supplies. If you're enrolled in Medicare, you pay a monthly premium based on your income. You have a small deductible that you must pay before Medicare Part B kicks in. And Medicare may pay a certain percentage, say 80 percent, for medical services and supplies.

For people with diabetes, Medicare Part B is really important. It covers blood glucose meters and control solution, test strips, lancets, and lancet devices. People who use insulin may qualify for up to 300 test strips and 300 lancets and people who do not use insulin may qualify for up to 100 test strips and 100 lancets every 3 months. Insulin pumps and supplies are also covered under Medicare Part B. You may need a provider's written authorization for some equipment or more of certain supplies.

Medicare Part B covers preventative care like tests for diabetes, cardiovascular disease, obesity, and glaucoma. It also covers diabetes education, medical nutrition education, and, sometimes, therapeutic shoes. Ask about the "Welcome to Medicare" physical exam and "Annual Wellness Visit" as part of your Medicare plan.

In 2013, Medicare started a National Mail-Order Program for Diabetic Testing Supplies for people who want supplies delivered to their homes. You have to use a Medicare contract supplier if you want home delivery of your supplies. You can still buy your testing supplies at retail pharmacies and stores. Please make sure that your store accepts "Medicare Assignment." You'll pay the same whether you order through the mail or buy from a store, because Medicare specifies that retailers can't charge more than your unmet deductible or 20 percent coinsurance.

DIABETES SUPPLIES AND SERVICES COVERED BY MEDICARE PART B

- Blood glucose meters and control solution.
- Blood glucose test strips.
- Lancets and lancet devices.
- Insulin pumps and insulin that the device uses.
- Therapeutic footwear and shoe inserts if ordered.
- Foot exam every 6 months.
- Glaucoma test every year.
- A1C tests.
- Flu and pneumococcal shots.
- Diabetes education (10 hours first year after diagnosis, 2 hours following years).
- Medical nutrition therapy as prescribed by your doctor.
- "Welcome to Medicare" preventative visit and yearly "Wellness" visit.

Medicare Part C

Medicare Part C, also called Medicare Advantage, covers *hospital* **and** *medical* **care.** You buy a Medicare Advantage plan from a private insurance company that has contracted with the government. Medicare Advantage plans are designed to cover services under original Medicare Parts A and B, but they sometimes cover prescription drugs and other services. Private insurers sell Medicare Advantage plans so they offer different plans and premiums. If you are considering enrolling in a Medicare Advantage plan, be sure to check its coverage for diabetes care, medications, and supplies. State Health Insurance Assistance Program (SHIP) counselors are able to assist you in selecting a Medicare Advantage plan. Visit https://shipnpr.acl.gov/ to find the SHIP in your state.

Medicare Part D

Medicare Part D covers prescription drugs. You buy Part D from a private insurance company approved by Medicare, so coverage varies from plan to plan. It is available to any Medicare-eligible person. Medicare Part D covers part of the cost of prescription drugs such as blood glucose pills, as well as some supplies like syringes, pens, needles, gauze, and alcohol swabs. It also covers insulin that isn't used in an insulin pump (Medicare B covers insulin used in a pump).

Each plan offers different coverage for medications and supplies, called a formulary, so you'll want to compare plans. For example, a plan may cover Amaryl, but not Glucotrol. See which plans offer the best coverage for your brands and make a chart to compare your costs. Most plans will have a monthly premium, but you may also have a deductible. SHIP counselors are able to assist you in selecting a Part D or Medicare Advantage plan. Visit https://shipnpr.acl.gov/ to find the SHIP in your state.

Most Medicare Part D plans have coverage gaps, also called the donut hole. Once you and the plan have spent a certain amount on your medications and supplies, you will be responsible for paying a large chunk of the cost. For example, in 2015, once you and the plan have spent $2,960 on covered medications, you pay 45 percent of the cost for brand-name medications and 65 percent of the cost for generic medications for the rest of the year. However, once your drug costs have reached $4,700—which includes the full cost of your drugs during the coverage gap, not just the portion you pay—you will be out of the coverage gap and will only pay as much as 5% of the cost for your prescriptions for the rest of the year. As part of the Affordable Care Act, consumers pay a smaller and smaller proportion of the costs in the coverage gap each year through 2020 when the gap will no longer exist.

EXTRA HELP IS AVAILABLE!

If you have limited income and resources, you may be able to qualify for a program called Extra Help to pay your prescription drug coverage costs. People who qualify may be able to get their prescriptions filled and pay little or nothing out of pocket. You can apply for Extra Help at any time. There's no cost to apply for Extra Help, so you should apply even if you're not sure if you qualify. To apply online, visit socialsecurity.gov/i1020. Or, call Social Security at 1-800-772-1213 to apply by phone or to get a paper application.

You do not have to enroll in Part D; you should compare Part D coverage with the coverage in Medicare Parts A and B or a Medicare Advantage Plan for your diabetes medications and supplies and other prescription drugs.

DIABETES SUPPLIES AND SERVICES USUALLY COVERED BY MEDICARE PART D

- Blood glucose medications.
- Syringes, needles, and alcohol swabs.
- Insulin (not given through a pump).
- Inhaled insulin devices and insulin used in those devices.

Keep in mind, for a Part D plan you'll have a separate premium, copayment, or coinsurance, and possibly a deductible.

Medigap

Medigap plans cover the extra costs of Medicare Parts A and B such as co-payments, co-insurance, and deductibles. You buy a Medigap plan from a private insurance company that must follow state and federal laws. Most states require that Medigap plans follow a standardized system of coverage so that you can compare the costs of plans offered by different insurers. You'll pay a monthly premium for your Medigap plan, in addition to your monthly premium for Part B.

For more information about Medigap, visit www.medicare.gov or call 1-800-MEDICARE.

OTHER HEALTH INSURANCE WITH MEDICARE

Your former employer may offer a "retiree" health insurance plan. A retiree health insurance plan usually has a monthly premium and covers the extra costs of Medicare to lower your out-of-pocket costs.

You can download or request a copy of "Choosing a Medigap Policy: A Guide to Health Insurance for People with Medicare." In addition, SHIP counselors may be able to assist you in selecting a Medigap plan. Visit https://shipnpr.acl.gov/ to find the SHIP in your state.

Medicaid and CHIP

Medicaid and the Children's Health Insurance Program (CHIP) cover certain medical and hospital costs for parents, pregnant women, children, seniors, and people with disabilities. Both are run by your state government and the coverage varies from state to state. However, all states are required to cover certain costs such as hospital visits, physician services, laboratory tests and x-rays, and long-term care such as nursing facilities.

The Affordable Care Act expanded Medicaid coverage to more people, although each state is responsible for providing this expanded coverage. Check healthcare.gov or call your state Medicaid office to find out if your state has expanded Medicaid. You may be newly eligible, depending on your circumstances or income. You can apply for Medicaid or CHIP at any time of the year and coverage begins immediately.

CHIP provides low-cost health care for children in families whose incomes are too high to qualify for Medicaid, but who can't afford private insurance. CHIP is administered by your state and coverage and costs vary from state to state. Visit insurekidsnow.gov or call 1-877-543-7669 to see if your children qualify.

Health Insurance for Veterans and Military Personnel

The U.S. Department of Veterans Affairs provides health care benefits for veterans, so visit www.va.gov or call 1-877-222-VETS to see if you qualify. Active duty service members, National Guard and Reserve members, retirees, their families and survivors may qualify for a health care program called TRICARE. To find out about eligibility, plans and coverage for diabetes medication and supplies, visit www.tricare.mil.

Individual Health Insurance

You may need to purchase your own health insurance if you don't have access to job-based health insurance or you don't qualify for Medicare or other programs. Before the Affordable Care Act, it was difficult for people with diabetes to find affordable health insurance because insurers could charge higher premiums or deny coverage due to a pre-existing condition of diabetes. Now, people purchasing their own health insurance have two options: buy a plan on a health insurance marketplace or buy a plan directly from a private insurance company.

Affordable Care Act: New Protections for Individual Plans

- Coverage for Young Adults: You can stay on your parent's plan until you're 26 as long as it covers dependents.
- Coverage for People with Diabetes: Since 2014, new individual plans are not allowed to deny coverage or charge more because a person has diabetes or any other pre-existing condition. Also, these plans cannot exclude coverage for treatment of diabetes or another pre-existing condition.
- Essential Health Benefits: Since 2014, a minimum set of "Essential Health Benefits" like hospitalization, prescription drugs, preventative services, and chronic disease management must be covered in all new individual and small group plans, including all plans sold in health insurance marketplaces.
- Summary of Benefits and Coverage: Individuals have the right to get a plain-language summary of a plan's benefits, called a Summary of Benefits and Coverage, or SBC. Plans must provide an SBC when a person is shopping for coverage, when there is a major change in benefits, or any time a person asks for it.

Courtesy: diabetes.org

HEALTH INSURANCE MARKETPLACE

You can buy an individual or family plan in a health insurance marketplace, sometimes called an exchange. The marketplace is run by your state, although some states have opted for the federal government to run their marketplaces. Typically, consumers will visit their state's health insurance marketplace website, although assistance is also available on the phone or in person. Visit healthcare.gov to find your state's health insurance marketplace.

In the marketplace, you can fill out an application to compare, choose, and enroll in a health insurance plan. Filling out an application will automatically tell you if you qualify for a program such as Medicaid or CHIP. It will also tell you if you qualify for financial assistance purchasing health insurance because of your income or circumstances, such as your employer not offering affordable health insurance plans. With this knowledge, you can begin shopping for health insurance. Keep in mind: coverage for diabetes medications, supplies, and services varies from plan to plan, so check to see if your brands and supplies are listed. You may also want to check if your preferred health care providers participate in the plan. Visit https://localhelp.healthcare.gov/ or call 1-800-318-2596 to find local assistance applying, choosing, and enrolling in marketplace coverage.

You have an annual enrollment period in the fall and winter in which you can sign up for a plan in the marketplace before coverage begins the following January. Certain life events such as a job loss or the birth of a child may allow you to sign up for a plan or make changes outside the enrollment period. Visit healthcare.gov or call 1-800-318-2596 to learn more about consumer protections under the Affordable Care Act.

PLANS DIRECTLY PURCHASED FROM INSURERS

You can also buy a health insurance plan directly from an insurer in most states. You'll have the same protections, such as nondiscrimination for pre-existing conditions and coverage for essential benefits, as plans purchased in the marketplace. However, you won't be eligible for financial assistance if you buy directly. Just like any plan, check to see if your preferred medications, diabetes supplies, services, and providers are covered.

14 Questions to Ask about Your Health Insurance

1. Are visits to my diabetes care provider covered?
2. Is there a limit on how many times I can see my diabetes care provider in a year?
3. How much will I have to pay per visit?
4. How much will the plan pay for a hospital stay?
5. Is there a limit on what I pay each year?
6. Is there a limit on what the plan pays each year?
7. When does coverage begin?
8. Does the plan cover blood glucose meters, strips, insulin, syringes, pens, pumps, or other supplies? Which brands?

9. Does the plan cover diabetes education?
10. Does the plan cover dietitians, mental health professionals, and specialists?
11. Which prescriptions are covered? What is the co-pay? And is there a prescription plan to reduce costs?
12. How often can prescriptions be refilled?
13. Is home health care covered? Any limitations?
14. Is long-term care covered?

NEXT UP

Your wellness depends on affordable, good health care. Your health care team, especially your diabetes care provider, can be one of your greatest assets in managing your diabetes. And you, the patient, are essential in everything from putting together a team, educating yourself through diabetes self-management education programs, and making the most of your doctor's visits. It's important to stay on top of changes in the health insurance marketplace—especially as they relate to your diabetes medications and supplies.

Next, you'll learn about navigating diabetes in the world beyond health care. In the upcoming chapter, discover your protections in the workplace and consider your options in discussing diabetes with your employer. Find out how to plan for travel—from airport security to travel overseas. Lastly, consider talking openly with your family members about your diabetes to prevent or delay *their* risk of diabetes in the future.

Chapter 8

Work, Travel, and Family

So far, you've learned the nuts and bolts of taking care of your body and mind. But how will you actually live your life while managing diabetes? Life can be unpredictable and managing your blood glucose can be unpredictable too. It's especially true when you're in a different environment like airport security or an unexpected circumstance like a low blood glucose episode in the middle of a work meeting. Give yourself a break. And know that doing your best comes with both ups and downs in terms of managing your diabetes.

In this chapter, find tips for navigating specific circumstances such as work, travel, and your family and home life. The work section describes some laws that protect you from discrimination. The travel section contains tips for travel, including the latest TSA guidelines for getting through airport security with your diabetes medications and supplies. The family section describes how healthy lifestyle habits at home can protect your whole family from the risk of type 2 diabetes.

WHAT'S INSIDE:

- Work
- Travel
- Family

WORK

Perhaps your first question is: Do I have to tell my employer or co-workers that I have diabetes? The most simple answer is, no. Whether you decide to discuss your diabetes at work is a personal matter. In the following section, you'll learn about your rights as a worker with diabetes, so that you can make an informed decision about discussing and managing your diabetes at work.

Your Rights on the Job

Disability laws protect people with diabetes in the workplace. At first, it may be hard to think of yourself as someone with a disability. However, having a disability, such as diabetes, can protect you from discrimination. Under the law, a disability is defined as a mental or physical impairment that substantially limits one or more major life activities, such as eating, walking, seeing, or caring for oneself, or a major bodily function such as endocrine function. Several laws, including the recently enacted Americans with Disabilities Act Amendments Act, protect people with disabilities.

Federal and State Anti-Discrimination Laws

- Americans with Disabilities Act: Protects employees against discrimination by private employers, labor unions, employment agencies, and state and local governments. The act does not apply to employers with fewer than 15 workers.
- Rehabilitation Act of 1973: Protects employees against discrimination by the executive branch of federal government and employers that receive federal money.
- Americans with Disabilities Act Amendments Act: Amends the Americans with Disabilities Act and Rehabilitation Act of 1973 by making it clear that people with conditions such as diabetes are protected from discrimination in the workplace.
- Congressional Accountability Act: Protects employees of Congress and most legislative branches.

  All states have their own anti-discrimination laws and agencies responsible for enforcing those laws. Some state anti-discrimination laws provide more comprehensive protection than do the federal laws.

Courtesy: diabetes.org

Under anti-discrimination laws, your employer cannot discriminate against you if you are qualified for the job and if you can do the job with or without "reasonable accommodation." Accommodation means that your employer makes changes in your work, work area, or schedule or provides equipment or training to help you do the job. The employer is required to make accommodations unless it would cause an "undue hardship" because it is very difficult or expensive to do.

FAMILY AND MEDICAL LEAVE ACT

Under the law, you may be entitled to 12 weeks of unpaid leave per year to deal with your own or a close family member's diabetes care. The leave can be taken in small blocks of time.

Discrimination at work can occur in almost any area of employment, including application procedures, hiring, training benefits, promotions, tenure, leaves of absence, layoffs, and firings. If you suspect discrimination, call the ADA at 1-800-DIABETES and ask for legal assistance to understand your rights or file a complaint or lawsuit.

Talking about Diabetes at Work

Although it's a personal decision, you have several advantages to talking about your diabetes at work. Being open about your diabetes can show others that people with diabetes are safe and responsible workers. If you take insulin, it may help if your co-workers know how to recognize, and perhaps treat, low blood glucose. Also, if you need to make changes in your schedule because of your diabetes, your employer may be more understanding of your needs.

Another important reason to tell your employer and co-workers about your diabetes is that this is the only way your employment rights will be protected by the Americans with Disabilities Act. Unless your employer knows about your diabetes, you won't be able to prove that the employer discriminated against you because of this disability.

Looking for a Job

You don't have to tell a potential employer that you have diabetes. However, if you decide to talk about diabetes during your interview, emphasize the positive. Refer to any awards you've won in previous jobs or other examples of your hard work and exemplary skills. If you haven't used much sick leave, point that out, too.

Keep in mind that a potential employer does not have to give you preference over other equally qualified people who apply for the job. The employer can choose whoever they feel can best perform a job.

Some professionals such as fire fighters, police officers, and commercial drivers are no longer subject to blanket bans that disqualify people with disabilities from these jobs. Instead, these professions may have specific guidelines or certification in which a candidate's blood glucose management and safety record is evaluated on an individual basis. Pilots with diabetes may not operate commercial planes and most branches of the military won't allow you to enlist if you have type 1 or type 2 diabetes.

A potential employer cannot ask you about your health or make you get a physical exam before offering you a job. Some employers require potential employees to have a physical exam once they've been made an offer and before they start the job. Some employers will require a physical exam if they think there are performance or safety issues related to your diabetes. These exams should be given by a health professional with expertise in diabetes. Call the American Diabetes Association at 1-800-DIABE-TES if you have questions or concerns about a physical exam at work.

TRAVEL

Travel can relax your mind and reinvigorate your soul. You may be planning a big trip to Europe or a weekend getaway. Whatever your plans, you should not let your diabetes keep you from travel. You can go anywhere you want to go. It just takes planning to manage your blood glucose while you're away from home. How you prepare will depend on where you're going, how you're getting there, and how long you will be there.

Planning Ahead

You'll want to make sure you're in good health before you take a trip. Consider visiting your health care provider for an exam and to discuss any questions that you have about managing your trip. Your health care provider can help you troubleshoot any emerging health concerns.

Your provider can write a letter about your diabetes that you carry with you when you travel. A doctor's letter should: state that you have diabetes, list your medications (pills, insulin, other injectables), and list equipment such as a blood glucose meter, insulin pen, needles, insulin pump, or continuous glucose monitor. It might also include your allergies or adverse reactions to food and medications. A doctor's letter can come in handy with airport security or when you're traveling in a foreign country.

Bring extra medication and testing supplies because it's better to have too much than not enough when your travel. Ask for a prescription for your medications (pills, insulin, or other injectables), insulin pens, or insulin pump. You'll have the prescription on hand if anything unexpectedly happens to your medication, or supplies. Even if you don't need a prescription in your state, you may need one in another state or foreign countries.

If you wear an insulin pump, call your pump company and ask for a loaner pump for your trip in case something happens to your pump while you're traveling.

Buy a medical ID bracelet or necklace that indicates that you have diabetes and wear it at all times while traveling.

Potential Packing List for Travel

- Letter from your provider stating you have diabetes.
- Written prescription for your medications and supplies.
- Medications such as insulin, pills, or other injectables.
- Syringes or pens for injectable medications.
- Insulin pump and pump supplies, if used.
- Glucose meter and test strips.
- Lancets or lancet devices.
- Glucose tablets or gel.
- Snacks and water.

Car Travel

Car travel can make it easier to follow your usual plan for meals, medications, and monitoring of blood glucose. Consider bringing a cooler with you so that you can pack your favorite meals and snacks in the car. Eating healthy on the road can be challenging, but try to seek out nutritious options. Also, find tips for eating out in Chapter 3.

Keep your insulin safe by protecting it from extreme heat or cold. In the summer, keep insulin in an insulated container with an ice pack or use a specially designed pack such as FRIO. Your car's glove compartment and trunk can get too hot for medications. Backpacks and cycle bags can also get quite hot in direct sunlight.

Air Travel

Traveling by airplane requires some extra planning. With increased airport security, you may need more time to ensure you make it to your plane on time and protect your supplies.

Always pack your diabetes medications and supplies in a carry-on bag—just in case your checked luggage gets lost. Keep in mind, your checked baggage may be put in extremely hot or cold storage areas of the plane that could damage medications.

It may take some extra steps to get through security with your diabetes medications and supplies. The ADA and Transportation Security Administration (TSA) have worked together to provide guidelines for traveling with these supplies. You can visit the ADA's website for more information or call the TSA Cares Help Line prior to traveling at 1-855-787-2227.

Remember the "no liquids over 3.4 ounces rule"? It DOES NOT apply to your medications. So you can bring liquid and gel medications such as insulin, Symlin, Byetta, and glucagon in any size container. Take the containers out of your carry-on bag and tell the TSA officer that these are your diabetes medications and supplies.

Items Permitted through Airport Security

- Insulin and insulin-loaded dispensing products (vials or box of individual vials, jet injectors, biojectors, pens, infusers, and pre-loaded syringes).
- Unlimited number of unused syringes when accompanied by insulin or other injectable medication.
- Lancets, alcohol swabs, blood glucose meters, test strips, control solution.
- Insulin pump and insulin pump supplies (cleaning agents, batteries, plastic tubing, infusion kit, catheter, and needle). Must be accompanied by insulin.

- Glucagon emergency kit.
- Urine ketone test strips.
- Unlimited number of used syringes when transported in sharps disposal container or other similar hard-surface container.
- Sharps disposal containers or similar hard-surface disposal container for storing used syringes and test strips.
- Liquids or gels (water, juice, or liquid nutrition).
- Continuous glucose monitors.
- All diabetes-related medication, equipment, and supplies.

Courtesy: diabetes.org

If you need to inject insulin during your flight, remember to consider the time zone changes as you fly. Here is a rule of thumb: Eastward travel results in a shorter day, so you may need less insulin. On the other hand, westward travel results in a longer day, so you may need more insulin. If you have questions, bring your upcoming flight schedule to your appointment with your diabetes care provider and ask his or her advice. Also, pressure differences on the plane can make it more difficult to fill a syringe. You may consider using an insulin pen for in-flight doses.

Airport travel days may require tweaks to your schedule. For example, changes in your mealtimes, sleep patterns, or activity can affect your blood glucose. Monitoring your blood glucose while traveling will help you make informed decisions.

Expect that food choices can be limited on flights and delays may interrupt service. We've all had those seemingly endless moments waiting on the tarmac for a flight to take off or to park at the airport gate. Bring your own snacks, meals, and drinks in your carry-on bag so that you know what you're eating and have control over when you eat.

10 Tips for Airport Travel

1. Arrive at the airport 2–3 hours prior to flight.
2. Review TSA's website for travel updates.
3. Download My TSA mobile app.
4. Whenever possible, bring prescription labels for medication and medical devices (while not required by TSA, making them available could speed things up).

5. Consider printing out and bringing an optional TSA Disability Notification Card, downloadable at tsa.gov.
6. Pack medications in a separate clear, resealable bag in your carry-on-luggage. Remove and show them to security at screening.
7. Keep a quick-acting source of glucose to treat low blood glucose and a snack such as a nutrition bar.
8. Carry or wear medical identification and carry contact information for your physician.
9. Pack extra supplies.
10. Be patient with lines, delays, and screening procedures.

Courtesy: diabetes.org

Travel Abroad

Visit your diabetes care provider well before your trip so that you can make necessary preparations. You'll probably want to carry a provider's note about your diabetes and get prescription refills. Carrying extra medication and supplies is especially important when traveling abroad because foreign countries may not have the same formulas and equipment.

Check out the Centers for Disease Control website, cdc.gov, for the most up-to-date information on the countries you plan to visit. The CDC has information on vaccinations, travel restrictions, and health and safety tips. Try to prepare by getting special vaccinations well in advance of your trip so that you're not caught off guard if the vaccinations affect your blood glucose. Visit a travel clinic in your hometown to find out more.

It's a good idea to learn how to say, "I have diabetes" and "Where is the hospital?" in the languages of the areas you'll be visiting. Write the phrases down to carry with you. You can point to them if you have trouble pronouncing them.

Ask your health insurance company about coverage for medical expenses and treatments while abroad. Some insurance may only pay a portion of the costs. If you want more coverage, consider purchasing travel insurance.

FAMILY

Your family is unique—and probably much different than the family across the street or on the other side of the country. However, almost everyone is touched, in some way, by diabetes in this country. You may pick up this book because you've recently been diagnosed with type 2 diabetes. Or you may have a parent or aunt or uncle who has type 2 diabetes. You may have a teenager in your family who is overweight and at risk for developing diabetes.

Diabetes in Children and Teens

There are more and more children and teens with type 2 diabetes. Until recently, type 2 diabetes was mostly diagnosed in people 40 years and older. A recent study found the rate of type 2 diabetes in children and teenagers increased by 30 percent from 2001 to 2009.

Generally, children with type 2 diabetes are overweight and have a family history of diabetes. They may have also been exposed to diabetes in utero because their mothers had gestational diabetes. Experts say that obesity and less physical activity among youth contribute to the problem.

Diabetes at earlier ages brings up issues for the health of children and their families—but also of our society as a whole. For example, children with diabetes may have an increased risk for early complications and difficulty with treatments. Children with diabetes can also go on to have diabetes during their reproductive years, which may lead to more diabetes in future generations.

Just like in adults, lifestyle changes can go a long way in delaying or preventing type 2 diabetes in youth. Children and teens need to eat 6 or more servings of fruits and vegetables per day, drink water instead of sugary sodas or sports drinks, and limit fast food and other unhealthy snacks. They also need an hour or more of exercise every day and to limit screen time to less than 2 hours a day. As a parent or caregiver, you'll need to challenge children to get active and offer them healthy foods. Visit ADA's website for tips for parents and children on preventing type 2 diabetes.

Why Family Matters

Family has an important role in type 2 diabetes, for many reasons, such as genetics, obesity, and our lifestyle choices. For these same reasons, your family could be the place to start if you're hoping to make changes for yourself, your spouse, or your children.

First, diabetes runs in families because it's genetic. Scientists don't yet know the specific genes or combination of genes that cause type 2 diabetes. However, scientists know that people with family members who have diabetes are more likely to have diabetes themselves.

Second, obesity tends to run in families too. Being overweight is a risk factor for type 2 diabetes and it can make blood glucose more difficult to manage. Everyone knows that inactivity and poor eating habits lead to obesity. Everyone knows that obesity is on the rise in America—at a startlingly fast rate, too.

Third—and this is the good news—healthy eating and exercise habits usually start at home with your family. People who make long-lasting healthy lifestyle choices don't make them in a bubble. Instead, they make healthy changes with their spouses, or with their children, or a friend. Support is one of the cornerstones of change.

Protecting Your Family from Type 2 Diabetes

- Talk about your food choices with your family and prepare nutritious family meals that everyone can enjoy.
- Involve your family in your education. Encourage them to visit your diabetes care provider, CDE, and dietitian.
- Make sure your family members have regular checkups with a provider experienced in diabetes. There are tests to detect markers for diabetes before it develops.
- Ask your family members to be your exercise partners. Set goals together and motivate one another.
- Work to achieve and maintain ideal weight for yourself and your children.
- Take the ADA Risk Test online at www.diabetes.org.

Share this book or an article online as an opener to talk about diabetes with your family. You may be surprised at your family's willingness to offer support, start exercising, and eat healthy foods. Or your actions could spark other family members to make healthy choices: today or even years down the road.

Resources

FOR MORE INFORMATION ON DIABETES

American Diabetes Association (National Office)
www.diabetes.org
1701 N. Beauregard Street
Alexandria, VA 22311
800-342-2383

Resources on diabetes basics, living with diabetes, and community events. Call or go online to receive free pamphlets, become a member, and subscribe to the monthly magazine *Diabetes Forecast*. Bookstore and ADA-hosted support groups also online.

National Institute of Diabetes and Digestive and Kidney Diseases
www.niddk.nih.gov
Bethesda, MD 20892
301-496-3583

Part of the National Institutes of Health, its website contains information for patients about diabetes care and research.

FOR THE VISUALLY CHALLENGED

American Council of the Blind
www.acb.org
2200 Wilson Boulevard, Suite 650
Arlington, VA 22201
202–467–5081 ● 800–424–8666

National information clearinghouse and legislative advocate that publishes a monthly magazine in Braille, large print, cassette, and computer disk versions.

American Foundation for the Blind
www.afb.org
2 Penn Plaza, Suite 1102
New York, NY 10121
212–502–7600 ● 800–232–5463

Works to establish, develop, and provide services and programs that assist visually challenged people in achieving independence.

American Printing House for the Blind
www.aph.org
1839 Frankfort Avenue
P.O. Box 6085
Louisville, KY 40206
502–895–2405 ● 800–223–1839

World's largest nonprofit organization creating educational, workplace, and independent living products and services for people who are visually impaired.

Lighthouse International
www.lighthouse.org
111 E. 59th Street
New York, NY 10022
(212) 821-9200 ● 800-829-0500

A national health association dedicated to fighting vision loss through prevention, treatment, and empowerment.

National Federation of the Blind
www.nfb.org
200 East Wells Street
Baltimore, MD 21230
410–659–9314

Membership organization providing information, networking, and resources. Some aids and appliances available through national headquarters. A division called the Diabetics Action Network provides resources for people with diabetes.

National Library Service (NLS) for the Blind and Physically Handicapped
www.loc.gov/nls
Library of Congress
1291 Taylor Street NW
Washington, DC 20542
202–707–5100 ● 202–707–0744 (TDD)

Through a national network of cooperating libraries, NLS administers a free library program of Braille and audio materials circulated to eligible borrowers.

Learning Ally
www.learningally.org
20 Roszel Road
Princeton, NJ 08540
800-221-4792

National nonprofit organization that is a leading provider of audiobooks for people with learning and reading disabilities.

The Seeing Eye, Inc.
www.seeingeye.org
10 Washington Valley Road
P.O. Box 375
Morristown, NJ 07963
973–539–4425

Offers guide dog training and instruction on working with a guide dog.

FOR AMPUTEES

Amputee Coalition
www.amputee-coalition.org
9303 Center Street, Suite 100
Manassas, VA 20110
888-267-5669

Nonprofit with mission to reach out and empower people affected by limb loss to achieve their full potential through education, support, and advocacy and to promote limb loss prevention.

National Amputation Foundation
www.nationalamputation.org
40 Church Street
Malverne, NY 11565
516–887–3600

Sponsor of *Amp-to-Amp* program, in which a new amputee is visited by an amputee who has resumed normal life. Provides information and educational materials.

TO FIND LONG-TERM OR HOME CARE

National Association for Home Care & Hospice (NAHC)
www.nahc.org
228 7th Street SE
Washington, DC 20003
202–547–7424

Largest trade association representing home care agencies and hospices. Offers free information for consumers about how to choose a home care agency, including searchable online directory of home care and hospice agencies.

TO FIND PHYSICIANS AND OTHER GENERAL HEALTH INFORMATION

American Association of Clinical Endocrinologists

www.aace.com
245 Riverside Avenue, Suite 200
Jacksonville, FL 32202
904-353-7878

Professional community of physicians specializing in endocrinology, diabetes and metabolism. Online directory of endocrinologists by area and endocrine focus.

American Board of Medical Specialties

www.abms.org
353 North Clark Street, Suite 1400
Chicago, IL 60654
312-436-2600

Record of physicians certified by 24 medical specialty boards. Directories of certified physicians organized by city of medical practice and alphabetically by physician names are available in many libraries and online.

American Medical Association

www.ama-assn.org
330 N. Wabash Avenue
Chicago, IL 60611
800–262-3211

Help in finding a doctor with online "DoctorFinder" and other educational resources for patients.

TO FIND DIABETES EDUCATORS AND DIETITIANS

American Association of Diabetes Educators

www.diabeteseducator.org
200 W. Madison Street, Suite 800
Chicago, IL 60606
800–338–3633

Resources for patients about diabetes education. Help in finding a diabetes educator, including searchable online directory.

Academy of Nutrition and Dietetics

www.eatright.org
120 South Riverside Plaza, Suite 2000
Chicago, IL 60606
800–877–1600

Nutrition information and help in finding a registered dietitian nutritionist in your area.

TO FIND MENTAL HEALTH PROFESSIONALS

American Association for Marriage and Family Therapy

www.aamft.org
112 South Alfred Street
Alexandria, VA 22314
703–838–9808

Offers a searchable online directory of marriage and family therapists across the country.

American Psychiatric Association

www.psych.org
1000 Wilson Boulevard, Suite 1825
Arlington, VA 22209
888-357-7924

Educational resources about mental health and listing of online locators for mental health professionals.

American Psychological Association

www.apa.org
750 First Street NE
Washington, DC 20002
202–336–5500 ● 800–374–2721

Educational resources for patients and online directory of psychologists.

National Association of Social Workers

www.socialworkers.org
750 First Street NE, Suite 700
Washington, DC 20002
202–408–8600

Oversees website www.helpstartshere.org, which offers resources for patients and features online directories to find a social worker.

American Association of Sexuality Educators, Counselors and Therapists (AASECT)

www.aasect.org
1444 I Street NW, Suite 700
Washington, DC 20005
202-449-1099

Online directory for sexuality educators, counselors, and therapists in your area.

TO FIND FOOT SPECIALISTS

American Podiatric Medical Association

www.apma.org
9312 Old Georgetown Road
Bethesda, MD 20814
301-581-9200

Online directory of podiatrists, as well as resources for patients, including section on diabetes awareness.

American Board of Foot and Ankle Surgery

www.abfas.org
445 Fillmore Street
San Francisco, CA 94117–3404
415–553–7800

Online directory of doctors who are board certified to practice foot and ankle surgery.

TO FIND EYE DOCTORS

American Optometric Association

www.aoa.org
243 N. Lindbergh Boulevard
St. Louis, MO 63141
800–365–2219

Information about eye and vision problems and taking care of your eyes. Online database of optometrists.

American Academy of Ophthalmology

www.aao.org
655 Beach Street
San Francisco, CA 94109

Mailing address:
P.O. Box 7424
San Francisco, CA 94120
415–561–8500

Oversees website www.geteyesmart.org, which has information about vision and eye health for patients. Also has online directory of ophthalmologists and "Ask an Eye M.D" service.

OTHER HELPFUL MEDICAL INFORMATION

U.S. Food and Drug Administration
Needles and Other Sharps (Safe Disposal)

http://www.fda.gov/MedicalDevices/ProductsandMedicalProcedures/
HomeHealthandConsumer/ConsumerProducts/Sharps/default.htm

Website with information about how to safely dispose of needles and other sharp devices.

MedicAlert Foundation

www.medicalert.org
2323 Colorado Avenue
Turlock, CA 95382
888–633–4298

Nonprofit organization offering access to emergency-support network through its MedicAlert memberships and IDs.

American Heart Association

www.heart.org
7272 Greenville Avenue
Dallas, TX 75231
800–242–8721

National organization devoted to fighting cardiovascular diseases and stroke. Website has resources about heart health and heart conditions.

National Kidney Foundation

www.kidney.org
30 E. 33rd Street
New York, NY 10016
800–622–9010

National organization dedicated to awareness, prevention, and treatment of kidney disease. Website includes information about kidney health and disease and being an organ donor. Publishes magazine for dialysis patients.

The Neuropathy Association
www.neuropathy.org
110 W. 40th Street, Suite 1804
New York, NY 10018
212-692-0662

Association providing neuropathy awareness, education, support, advocacy, and research. Online directory of neuropathy physicians and information about support groups.

American Chronic Pain Association
www.theacpa.org
P.O. Box 850
Rocklin, CA 95677
800-533-3231

Association offering support and education for pain management. Find a support group in your area or educational resources online.

FOR ORGAN DONATION

Donate Life America
www.donatelife.net
701 E. Byrd Street, 16th Floor
Richmond, VA 23219
804-377-3580

Not-for-profit alliance of national organizations and state teams across the United States committed to increasing organ, eye, and tissue donation. Register online to be a donor.

United Network for Organ Sharing
www.unos.org
P.O. Box 2484
Richmond, VA 23218
804–782–4800

Runs the Organ Procurement and Transplant Network for the federal government and oversees www.transplantliving.org, with information about organ transplants and donations.

FOR TRAVELERS

Centers for Disease Control and Prevention

www.cdc.gov/travel
1600 Clifton Road
Atlanta, GA 30333
800-232-4636

Provides travel health information for a variety of destinations and subject areas. Also publishes *CDC Health Information for International Travel* (also called the Yellow Book). Can order online or by calling 1-800-451-7556.

International Association for Medical Assistance to Travellers

www.iamat.org
1623 Military Road, #279
Niagara Falls, NY 14304
716–754–4883

Provides travelers with health information and access to a worldwide network of English-speaking doctors.

FOR FITNESS

Centers for Disease Control and Prevention
Division of Nutrition, Physical Activity and Obesity

www.cdc.gov/physicalactivity

Tips for healthy eating and active living, including information on state and community programs.

American College of Sports Medicine

www.acsm.org
401 W. Michigan Street
Indianapolis, IN 46202
317–637–9200

President's Council on Fitness, Sports & Nutrition

www.fitness.gov
1101 Wootton Parkway, Suite 560
Rockville, MD 20852
240-276-9567

A council of educators, athletes, chefs, physicians, and fitness professionals, appointed by the President, who promote programs to help Americans lead healthy lives.

FOR SENIORS

AARP

www.aarp.org
601 E Street, NW
Washington, DC 20049
888-687-2277

Largest membership organization in the nation, offering services from prescription drug plans to insurance and other discounts.

National Council on the Aging

www.ncoa.org
1901 L Street, NW, 4th floor
Washington, DC 20036
202–479–1200

Advocacy group concerned with developing and implementing high standards of care for the elderly.

U.S. Department of Health and Human Services Eldercare Locator

www.eldercare.gov
800-677-1116

A nationwide service that connects older Americans and their caregivers with information on senior services. A public service of HHS' Administration on Aging.

FOR EQUAL EMPLOYMENT INFORMATION

American Bar Association Commission on Disability Rights

www.americanbar.org/groups/disabilityrights
1050 Connecticut Avenue, NW, Suite 400
Washington, DC 20036
202-662-1000

Provides information and technical assistance on all aspects of disability law.

Disability Rights Education and Defense Fund

www.dredf.org
3075 Adeline Street, Suite 210
Berkeley, CA 94703
510–644–2555

Provides technical assistance and information to employers and individuals with disabilities on disability rights legislation and policies.

U.S. Equal Employment Opportunity Commission

www.eeoc.gov
131 M Street, NE
Washington, DC 20507
202–663–4900 ● 202–663–4494 (TTY)

Responsible for enforcing federal laws that make it illegal to discriminate against a job applicant or an employee because of a person's race, color, sex, national origin, age, disability, or genetic information.

FOR HEALTH INSURANCE INFORMATION

HealthCare.gov
www.healthcare.gov
800-318-2596 ● 855-889-4325 (TTY)

A federal government website managed by the U.S. Centers for Medicare and Medicaid Services that includes a health insurance marketplace where individuals and small businesses can shop for health coverage.

AARP Member Advantages
www.aarphealthcare.com
P.O. Box 1017
Montgomeryville, PA 18936
800-894-6032

The AARP administers a variety of health insurance plans: Medicare plans, health insurance, hospital insurance, and life insurance. Plans are available to people 50 and over. Not all plans are available in all areas.

Medicare Hot Line
www.medicare.gov
Centers for Medicare & Medicaid Services
7500 Security Boulevard
Baltimore MD 21244
800–633–4227 ● 877–486–2048 (TTY)

For information and various publications about Medicare.

Social Security Administration

www.ssa.gov
Social Security Administration
Office of Public Inquiries
1100 West High Rise
6401 Security Boulevard
Baltimore, MD 21235
800–772–1213 ● 800–325–0778 (TTY)

For information and various publications about Social Security. Find your local SSA office online.

Robert Wood Johnson Foundation

www.rwjf.org
Route 1 and College Road East
P.O. Box 2316
Princeton, NJ 08543
877-843-7953

An independent philanthropic foundation working to improve the health and health care of Americans. Online tools covering health insurance and other aspects of health costs.

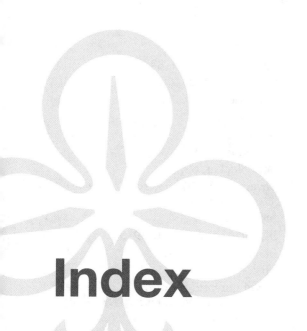

Index

Note: Page numbers in **bold** indicate an in-depth discussion.

A

A1C, 4–5, 10, 101
Academy of Nutrition and Dietetics, 96–97
acarbose, 59
accommodation, 123
Accountable Care Organizations, 95
ACE inhibitor, 69, 73, 78
acesulfame potassium, 34
activity tracker, 45
aerobic exercise, 45–46
Affordable Care Act (ACA), 95, 108–110, 114, 116–118
Afrezza, 67
African American population, 6
age, 5
airport security, 125–126
air travel, 126–128
albiglutide, 61
albumin, 79–80
alcohol, 23, 32–33
alcohol-free medication, 21

alogliptin, 58
alpha-glucosidase inhibitor, 59
American Association of Diabetes Educators, 96, 101–102
American Cancer Society, 52
American College of Sports Medicine, 98
American Diabetes Association
    air travel, 126
    blood glucose recommendations, 13
    blood pressure recommendations, 68
    diabetes education, 101–102
    discrimination, 123
    emotional health resources, 91
    eye exam recommendations, 99
    foot exam recommendations, 99
    MyFoodAdvisor, 51
    parents and children, tips for, 129
    physical activity recommendations, 47
    physical exam at work, 124